Lung Cancer

A Guide to Diagnosis and Treatment

Second Edition

Walter J. Scott, M.D.

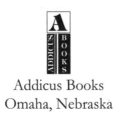

Addicus Books
Omaha, Nebraska

An Addicus Nonfiction Book

ISBN 978-1-886039-09-4
Interior design by Jack Kusler
Illustrations by Jack Kusler

This book is not intended to be a substitute for a physician, nor do the authors intend to give advice contrary to that of an attending physician.

Library of Congress Cataloging-in-Publication Data

Scott, Walter, 1954-
    Lung cancer : a guide to diagnosis and treatment / Walter J. Scott. -- 2nd ed.
        p. cm.
    Includes index.
    ISBN 978-1-886039-09-4 (pbk.)
1. Lungs--Cancer--Popular works. I. Title.
RC280.L8S36 2011
616.99'424--dc23

                                              2011042503

Addicus Books, Inc.
P.O. Box 45327
Omaha, Nebraska 68145
www.AddicusBooks.com

Printed in the United States of America
10 9 8 7 6 5 4 3 2 1

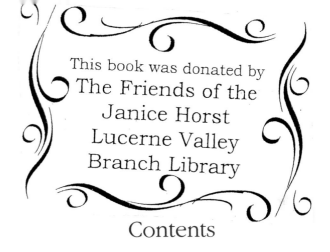

Contents

Acknowledgments

This book would not have been possible without the efforts of a great many people. Most importantly, I wish to express my gratitude to my patients and their families. Their willingness to share their personal experiences with me has been a source of inspiration and renewal.

I also wish to thank the members of the Fox Chase Cancer Center Multidisciplinary Thoracic Service and the rest of the staff at Fox Chase Cancer Center, in Philadelphia, for their commitment to improving care for patients with lung cancer. Thanks also to the medical students, residents, and fellows at Fox Chase for their hard work and tough questions.

I am grateful for the support of Rod Colvin and Jack Kusler of Addicus Books. Their patience and guidance throughout the preparation of the manuscript have helped make this a much more useful book.

I thank Addison Tolentino, M.D., medical oncologist and co-author of *Colon and Rectal Cancer*, for his help with the chapter on chemotherapy. I also thank Carol Kornmehl, M.D., radiation oncologist and author of *The Best News about Radiation Therapy*, for her contribution to the chapter on radiation therapy. In addition, I thank Mark Pool, M.D., laboratory medical director at Riverside Medical Center, in Kankakee, Illinois, for his help with the development of this book.

Finally, a special thanks goes to my wife, Christine Beardmore, M.A., a psychotherapist, for her help with the chapter on emotional support.

Introduction

If you are reading this book, you or someone you care about has probably been diagnosed with lung cancer. Over the years, many of my patients have told me that, after their diagnosis, they were overwhelmed by the sheer number of medical tests, procedures, and treatments they had to undergo. It is my intention in writing this book to take away some of the fear of the unknown and provide you with answers to the pressing questions you have about your diagnosis and treatment.

If you have been diagnosed with lung cancer, your survival and your quality of life depend on understanding your options and making sure you receive the best available treatment. Thanks to new treatments and new combinations of treatments, thousands of men and women survive lung cancer each year. My wish is that you will receive the best possible treatment so that you can improve your chances of becoming a lung cancer survivor.

—Walter J. Scott, M.D., F.A.C.S.

1 Lung Cancer: An Overview

Hasn't it seemed that cancer was always something that happened to someone else? But now, you or perhaps a loved one has been diagnosed with lung cancer. Your initial reaction may have been shock or that feeling of dread that comes with having your worst fears confirmed. You may feel sad, confused, and scared. These are normal reactions.

After receiving the initial diagnosis, you may have wondered what happens next? What medical tests will you undergo? What treatment will you need? Hopefully, the chapters that lie ahead will answer many of your questions. To start, however, this first chapter will give you a basic understanding of lung cancer.

How Lung Cancer Develops

Cancer is a collection of cells growing out of control. The cells in our bodies are constantly growing, and each cell contains a set of instructions, like software in a computer, that regulate cell behavior. Sometimes, a change, or *mutation*, occurs in a cell's growth pattern. When these mutations continue to occur—as many as ten to twenty may be required—the once-normal cells begin to grow abnormally. These new growths are called cancers.

Lung cancer usually arises from the cells that line the airways and the nearby mucous glands. When the airways are exposed to toxins we inhale, the transformation of normal cells to cancer begins with a condition called *hyperplasia*—an increase in the number of cells lining one part of the airways

Lung Anatomy

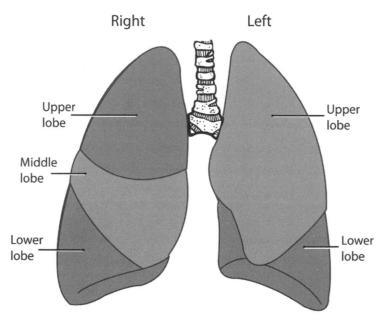

Each lung is divided into lobes. The right lung has three lobes—upper, middle, and lower. The left lung has two lobes—upper and lower.

through which we breathe. This is followed by the development of *dysplasia*, which is an increase in the number of abnormal cells that line the airways. From this point, malignant cells can emerge. If left untreated, these cells can continue to grow and invade surrounding tissues.

How Lung Cancer Spreads

There are three ways cancer can spread: into surrounding tissues from the original tumor, through the blood, or through lymph nodes. The lymph nodes are part of the body's immune system—they filter the blood for foreign particles, such as bacteria or cancer cells. There are hundreds of lymph nodes throughout your body. Normally, when not inflamed or cancerous, lymph nodes are the size of raisins. Lung cancer can spread to lymph nodes in the chest.

In addition to spreading to lymph nodes, the malignant cells can escape into the bloodstream and travel throughout the body. Lung cancer most commonly spreads to the liver, but can also spread to the bones, bone marrow, brain, and adrenal glands. When a secondary cancer forms in any of these organs, it is called a *metastasis.*

Types of Lung Cancer

There are more than a dozen types of lung cancer, but more than about 90 percent of them fall into two main categories: *non-small cell lung cancer* and *small cell lung cancer.* These two forms of lung cancer grow differently and are also treated differently. Whether the cancer is non-small cell or small cell is determined by the size and other characteristics of the cancer cells as they appear when viewed through a microscope.

Non-Small Cell Lung Cancer

Approximately 80 percent of all lung cancers fall into the category of non-small cell lung cancer. It's called non-small cell because when viewed through a microscope, the cells appear large—or non-small. There are two main forms of non-small cell lung cancer: *adenocarcinoma* and *squamous cell carcinoma.*

Adenocarcinomas are usually found in the outer edges of the lung and arise from the tiny glands that produce mucus in the smaller airways (called *alveoli*). This is the most common form of non-small cell lung cancer.

Squamous cell carcinomas generally arise in the bronchial tubes in the center of the chest. These cancers grow in the squamous cells in the bronchial lining.

Small Cell Lung Cancer

About 13 percent of all lung cancers are categorized as small cell lung cancer. This form of lung cancer often occurs in the lining of the major breathing tubes in the center of the chest. Small cell lung cancer tends to grow quickly. By the time

Normal Cells

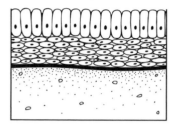

Normal cells line the airways. The cells are similar in shape and grow in an orderly fashion.

Precancerous Cells

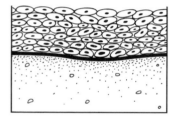

The cells in the top layer are flattened, becoming abnormal. The change in cell structure can be caused by pollutants, such as tobacco.

Cancer

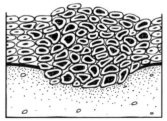

Cells change into cancer cells, form a mass, and begin to destroy surrounding tissue.

it is diagnosed, it has often spread to the lymph nodes in the center of the chest and may even have spread through the bloodstream to other organs in the body.

Risk Factors for Lung Cancer

Most experts believe that more than 80 percent of all cancers occur in response to environmental factors. These factors include such things as cigarette smoke and toxic chemicals. Other risk factors include aging and heredity may also be factors.

Cigarette Smoking

Cigarette smoke contains some four thousand chemicals, and at least fifty of them are known *carcinogens* (cancer-producing substances). Although fewer than 20 percent of smokers will develop lung cancer, scientists have determined that the chemicals in cigarette smoke cause more than 80 to 90 percent of all lung cancers. The risk of developing lung cancer increases significantly with ten to twenty years of regularly smoking one to two packs of cigarettes per day.

For smokers who do not develop lung cancer, smoking may still take a toll on their health in other ways. Many thousands will develop, and die prematurely from, illnesses such as emphysema, chronic obstructive pulmonary disease (COPD), heart disease, stroke, and accelerated hardening of the coronary arteries, which can lead to heart attacks.

Quitting smoking decreases a person's risk of developing lung cancer. Ten years after quitting, the risk drops by half. Smoking's harmful effects on the heart also decrease immediately with smoking cessation.

Before 1930, the U.S. government kept few statistics on lung cancer because the disease was so rarely seen. However, by 1986, it had long been the leading cause of cancer deaths in American men and had surpassed breast cancer as the leading cause of cancer deaths in American women. How did lung cancer become the most common cause of death from cancer in both sexes? The main cause is the rise in cigarette consumption.

Passive Smoking

If you live with or are frequently around smokers, passive smoking may be a risk factor for you. Nonsmokers who live with smokers are estimated to have a 24 percent higher risk of developing lung cancer compared to those who do not live with smokers. Passive smoking claims nearly three thousand lives annually in the United States.

Environmental Pollution

Certain environmental factors are thought to increase the risk of developing lung cancer. The natural, odorless gas called *radon* is considered a carcinogen. Radon is believed to cause some twenty thousand lung cancer deaths annually in the United States, making it the second-leading cause of such deaths.

Radon is created by the radioactive decay of uranium and is found in soil and rocks. It may seep into homes and other buildings through pipes, drains, or cracks in foundations.

Asbestos, a fibrous mineral once commonly used in the construction of homes and other buildings, is considered the

**Lung Cancer
Statistics**

- Nearly 220,000 Americans are diagnosed with lung cancer each year.
- Lifetime risk of lung cancer for men: 1 in 13
- Lifetime risk of lung cancer for women: 1 in 16
- Average age at time of diagnosis: 71
- Only 3% of lung cancer patients are under age 45.
- Lung cancer is the leading cause of cancer deaths in men and women.

—American Cancer Society

cause of a form of cancer known as *mesothelioma*. Asbestos fibers may break into particles and float into the environment. When inhaled, the particles may stick to the lungs and remain there for a lifetime. The long-term effects of exposure to asbestos may not develop until twenty to thirty years after the exposure.

The risk of developing cancer from asbestos exposure is based on the amount and duration of the exposure. People who have worked around asbestos have a five times greater risk of developing lung cancer compared to those who have never worked around asbestos. People who have been exposed to asbestos and who have also been smokers have a risk fifty to ninety times greater than that of nonsmokers. In the 1970s, the U.S. government began banning the use of asbestos in the construction of homes and other buildings.

Other chemicals that increase the risk of lung cancer include *vinyl chloride*, an odorless gas used in the making of plastics and vinyl, and *chromium*, a metallic element used in chrome plating and stainless steel welding. Also associated with an increased risk of lung cancer is exposure to nickel refinery dust and fumes; nickel is used in the making of metals— most notably, stainless steel. Finally, exposure to arsenic may cause lung cancer; arsenic is found in pesticides and is used in the production of many products, including glass, enamel, and textiles.

Age

Increasing age lowers a person's defenses against virtually all diseases, including lung cancer. Nearly 70 percent of those diagnosed with lung cancer are over the age of sixty-five. Only about 3 percent of cases are diagnosed in people younger than forty-five.

Also, as we age we are more susceptible to the actions of free radicals, organic molecules that are responsible for aging, tissue damage, and possibly some diseases.

Heredity

Genetics do not appear to be a major risk factor in who develops lung cancer. However, research has shown that genes may play a role in some families. It is believed that some individuals may not be able to rid their bodies of certain cancer-causing agents, leaving them more vulnerable to cancer. Others may have faulty repair mechanisms in their cells, also leaving them at higher risk for cancer.

In Summary

Lung cancer is the second most common cancer among both men and women in the United States. Approximately 220,000 thousand Americans are diagnosed with lung cancer annually. The disease accounts for 15 percent of all new cancers and causes more deaths than cancers of the colon, prostate, and breast combined.

The key to surviving lung cancer is early detection. However, symptoms of lung cancer are not always noticeable, especially if the cancer is in at an early stage. The next chapter will discuss the symptoms of lung cancer.

2 Symptoms of Lung Cancer

The symptoms of lung cancer can be elusive. In fact, about 25 percent of lung cancer patients have no symptoms at all at the time of diagnosis; their cancer is caught during routine X-rays or scans, often to the surprise of both the patient and the doctor. In many cases, symptoms of lung cancer are not noticeable until the cancer has progressed.

If a person has symptoms that may be associated with lung cancer, his or her physician will consider the symptoms in relation to the person's history. For example, a doctor would not immediately suspect lung cancer in a twenty-five-year-old woman who has persistent coughing and wheezing. On the other hand, a diagnosis of lung cancer would be more likely in a sixty-five-year-old woman who has smoked two packs of cigarettes for thirty years and has the same symptoms.

It's important to seek medical attention when you have any of the symptoms of lung cancer. The sooner symptoms are reported, the sooner the problem, if any, can be diagnosed and treated.

Persistent Coughing

As noted in chapter 1, lung cancer usually arises from the cells lining the airways. The nerves lining the airways detect the presence of anything foreign—dust, dirt, blood, or a tumor. These nerves stimulate the cough reflex, designed to help the body rid itself of foreign particles and keep the airways clean. If a tumor develops in the large airways, coughing may be a prominent symptom. People with lung cancer who never complain of a cough probably have a tumor located away from the center of the lung, in the smaller airways, where there are few cough receptors.

Blood in the Sputum

Sputum refers to mucus coughed up from the lungs. If the surface of a tumor bleeds, the patient may cough up blood-tinged mucus. This serious symptom, called *hemoptysis,* should be evaluated immediately.

When breathing passages are blocked completely by a tumor, infection may occur in the blocked or obstructed area. This leads to fever and coughing up dark sputum. It is important not to confuse this condition with pneumonia, which produces similar symptoms but responds to antibiotic treatment.

Wheezing

A tumor may result in wheezing, the sound produced when air tries to pass through a partially blocked airway in the lung. A tumor will produce *localized wheezing*, best heard on the side of the chest where the tumor is located.

Chest Pain

The surface lining of the lungs and the inside lining of the chest cavity, known as the *pleura,* have many nerve fibers. Therefore, a cancer that irritates the surface linings of the lung or the chest wall can cause *chest pain.* The pain usually occurs where the cancer is irritating the pleura. It may be constant, or it may come and go with breathing. This pain is called *pleuritic chest pain.* It suggests that the cancer may be growing on the surface of the lung and even into the chest wall. If the cancer has invaded the surface of the lung or the chest wall, it is more advanced. However, sometimes the cancer may irritate the surface of the lung without actually growing into it. Often, surgery is the only way to find out exactly how far the cancer has spread.

Because lung tissue itself has no nerves that sense pain, cancer may grow to a large size within the lung without causing pain. This is one reason why lung cancer is difficult to diagnose in its early stages.

Persistent Hoarseness

The *laryngeal nerves* supply motor function to the vocal cords, allowing them to move, giving a person his or her normal voice. These nerves start in the brain, travel down into the chest, and then go back up into the neck to supply the voice box and vocal cords. Lung cancer may grow into one of these nerves where it passes through the chest. If this happens, the vocal cord controlled by the nerve becomes weakened or even paralyzed, and the person becomes hoarse. Persistent hoarseness or a change in the quality of a person's voice needs to be evaluated. A chest X-ray should be obtained as part of this evaluation.

Drooping Eyelid

If the cancer involves the sympathetic nerves, one of the eyelids may droop slightly or take longer to open than the other (*lid lag*). The sympathetic nerves, which control involuntary actions such as breathing, run in a chain along either side of the spine. These nerves are most vulnerable to damage from cancer arising in the top of the lung. Because the chest cavity narrows in this area, a cancer growing there may easily compress and grow into the surrounding structures.

In this case, a person may also have trouble seeing because one pupil is constricted (*miosis*), or he or she may notice that one side of the face is drier or less sweaty (*anhidrosis*). A combination of these symptoms is called *Horner's syndrome*.

Pain in the Arm and Armpit

Constant pain in the arm and armpit, typically accompanied by other symptoms, is known as *Pancoast syndrome*. The nerves that supply the arm and armpit come from the neck and travel over the top of the lung. A cancer in the top of the lung may compress these nerves, causing severe pain in the arm and armpit.

Shortness of Breath

Shortness of breath is a common symptom among people with lung cancer. Lung cancer can cause shortness of breath in several ways. A tumor that arises in a major airway and blocks the passage of air into an entire lung may cause shortness of breath. Lung cancer can also cause a buildup of fluid around the outside of the lung; this fluid buildup, called a *pleural effusion*, may prevent the lung from fully expanding, causing shortness of breath. Lung cancer may even affect the sac around the heart, known as the *pericardium*; it can cause fluid to build up within the sac, preventing the heart from working properly and resulting in shortness of breath.

Shortness of breath can also be caused by damage to the nerves in the diaphragm, a muscle important to breathing. If lung cancer involves one of these nerves, the half of the diaphragm that it controls becomes paralyzed. Movement of air in and out of the chest decreases, causing shortness of breath.

Swelling of the Face and Arms

Cancer arising in the right lung may compress the *superior vena cava*, the great vein that drains the blood from the head and arms and delivers it back to the heart and lungs. This compression can result in swelling of the face and arms, which is known as *superior vena cava syndrome*. This may prove serious if swelling in the neck and trachea interferes with breathing.

Neurological Symptoms

When lung cancer spreads to the central nervous system— the brain and spinal cord—headaches may occur. At first, they may seem no different from common tension headaches. Only when the headaches persist or become more severe do most people seek evaluation.

Other neurological symptoms include changes in alertness as well as nausea and vomiting not related to another cause. Less common symptoms include weakness (either generalized or in the extremities), loss of bowel or bladder control, and seizures.

Skeletal Pain

As noted in chapter 1, lung cancer can spread to bone. As a bone tumor grows, it destroys the surrounding bone, causing pain. Therefore, localized skeletal pain in someone suspected of having lung cancer should be evaluated with additional tests to determine if a metastasis is present. The most common sites for bone metastases are in the spine, the pelvic bones, and the femur (the large bone in the thigh).

Weight Loss and Fatigue

Symptoms such as unintentional weight loss and unexplained fatigue are called *nonspecific symptoms*—they are not specific to lung cancer and could have many causes. However, if these symptoms are present in a person suspected of having lung cancer, it would be a further indication of the disease.

Determining Cause of Symptoms

The symptoms described in this chapter can be caused by other ailments—they don't always indicate lung cancer. However, if you have these symptoms, it's important to be examined by your physician. If your doctor suspects lung cancer, he or she will want you to undergo diagnostic testing, which is discussed in the next chapter.

3 Getting a Diagnosis

If you have *any* of the symptoms of lung cancer, it's important that you see your doctor immediately. The earlier the diagnosis is made, the sooner treatment can begin. Early treatment improves your prospects of being cured.

However, a physician cannot make a diagnosis based on symptoms alone. A true diagnosis can be made only upon the completion of diagnostic testing. If, after conducting a thorough physical examination, your doctor suspects lung cancer, he or she may order any of a number of tests to determine whether cancer is present.

Diagnostic Tests

Chest X-ray

An ordinary chest X-ray is still the most common imaging study performed when symptoms or a physical examination suggest disease in the chest. The discovery of a mass in the lung is the most common chest X-ray finding in a person with lung cancer. The chest X-ray may also detect an abnormal widening of the area between the lungs. Such an abnormal contour may indicate the presence of a tumor or lymph nodes that have enlarged as the result of a tumor.

If your physician detected a growth in a previous lung X-ray, he or she can review new chest X-rays to check the size of the growth. If it has not grown or changed as shown by chest X-rays obtained over at least a two-year period, the chance of the growth being a cancer is less than 5 percent.

Chest X-rays may also show signs of pneumonia, fluid

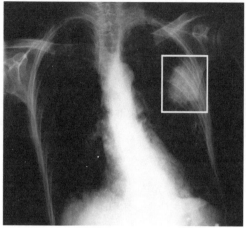

This lung X-ray shows a 71-year-old man with lung cancer in the left lung.

around the lungs, or abnormalities in the bones.

Computerized Tomography

A *computerized tomography (CT) scan* is also known as a *computerized axial tomography (CAT) scan*. A CT scan of the chest is standard for evaluating people with known or suspected lung cancer. A CT scan produces internal pictures of the body. A chest CT provides more detail and information than a chest X-ray does. It can confirm the presence of a tumor first seen on a chest X-ray and can better identify tumor characteristics, such as an irregular surface or calcification, a process in which calcium builds up and hardens.

Furthermore, a chest CT is much more accurate than a chest X-ray in identifying enlarged lymph nodes in the lungs or in the center of the chest. This is important because enlarged lymph nodes may contain metastatic lung cancer cells.

Positron Emission Tomography

A *positron emission tomography (PET) scan* is an imaging test similar to the chest X-ray and the CT scan; however, a PET scan reveals cell function, whereas the other tests show only cell structure.

A person undergoing a PET scan will first be given a glucose (sugar) solution intravenously. Cancer cells use glucose at a faster rate than normal cells do. If cancer is present, a tumor will show up in a PET scan, having absorbed the glucose solution. Generally, the more glucose the tumor absorbs, the more likely it is cancerous.

14

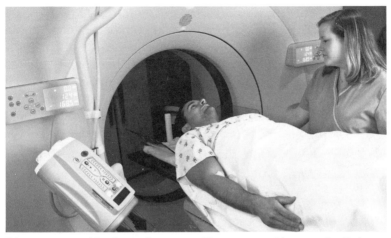

CT scans are used in diagnosing cancer. The scans provide more detail than a standard X-ray.

Magnetic Resonance Imaging

The *magnetic resonance imagining scan (MRI)* is a scan that uses a combination of powerful magnets, radio frequency, and computers to take pictures of your soft tissues, bones, and other internal body structures. In lung cancer patients, the MRI is often used to determine whether cancer has spread to the brain. It may be used to scan the chest to better determine the location of a tumor.

Because the MRI uses a powerful magnetic field, you cannot wear any metals such as jewelry, watches, or eyeglasses while undergoing the scan. You should not have an MRI if you have any metal screws, pins or plates in your body or if you have a pacemaker or cochlear ear implant.

Sputum Cytology

Sputum, as you many recall, is mucus coughed up from the lungs. *Cytology* refers to the study of cells. Sputum cytology involves collecting mucus coughed up by an individual and examining its cellular makeup under a microscope to check for malignant cells. The most accurate way to perform this test is to collect early-morning samples of sputum on three separate days.

Biopsies

Imaging studies can reveal important features about tumors, but they cannot provide absolute proof that cancer is present. Such a determination can be made only with a tissue analysis. This means doing a *biopsy*, which involves gathering a tissue sample from the tumor. A physician will choose from several methods to perform a biopsy depending on such factors as the likelihood that cancer is present and the size and location of the tumor.

Bronchoscopy

A *bronchoscopy* is a procedure that allows a physician to look inside a person's lungs using an illuminated tube called a *bronchoscope*. The bronchoscope is inserted through the mouth and then passed through the trachea and into the lungs. Since lung cancer often arises inside the airways, the physician performing the bronchoscopy will typically see a tumor located in the large air passages of the lungs. During the procedure, a biopsy can be performed and the tissue sample can be tested to determine whether the tumor is cancerous.

A bronchoscopy provides helpful information about the location and stage of the tumor and whether it can be completely removed with surgery. This procedure, however, is less successful in examining tumors located toward the edges of the lungs. A bronchoscopy can be performed without general anesthesia. Most people tolerate the procedure well.

Transthoracic Needle Aspiration

A *transthoracic needle aspiration (TTNA)* is another common method used to obtain a tumor sample. TTNA is used mostly to study tumors closer to the chest wall, as opposed to tumors that are more centrally located. The test is usually performed by a radiologist, a physician who specializes in using X-rays and imaging scans to diagnose disease.

After injecting a local anesthetic into the chest area, the radiologist uses a scanner to guide a needle through the chest wall and into the tumor. Cells from the tumor are suctioned into a syringe. A specially trained *pathologist*—a doctor who examines tissues and organs for diseases—then examines the cell samples under a microscope to check for malignancy.

TTNA can also be used to biopsy enlarged lymph nodes. The patient, however, must be able to cooperate by holding his or her breath during certain parts of the procedure.

TTNA is a relatively simple outpatient procedure and doesn't require a general anesthetic. However, one disadvantage of TTNA is that a certain number of patients will develop a collapsed lung (*pneumothorax*) when the needle passes through the lung. Most of the time, the collapsed lung will simply reexpand, but sometimes, a *chest tube* must be inserted between the ribs to reexpand the lung.

A more serious disadvantage of TTNA is that the needle sometimes misses the part of the tumor that contains the cancer cells; thus, the test might wrongly suggest that the tumor is benign. If the physician suspects that this may have occurred, he or she may order another biopsy using a different method or may recommend monitoring the tumor by performing another CT scan in several weeks; if the scan shows that the tumor has grown, cancer may be suspected.

Cervical Mediastinoscopy

This method is occasionally used to biopsy a tumor but is more often used to biopsy the *mediastinal lymph nodes*. These nodes are located toward the center of the chest, which is called the *mediastinum*. A *cervical mediastinoscopy* is a minimally invasive surgery in which a small incision is made directly over the trachea, just above the breastbone. A mediastinoscope—a small tube that the surgeon looks through—is inserted next to the trachea. With the mediastinoscope in place, the surgeon can insert another instrument through it and remove a piece of the tumor or enlarged lymph node.

For this procedure, the patient must be under general anesthesia; however, the procedure may be performed on an outpatient basis. The procedure is generally safe, but is underused because some surgeons are reluctant to perform it. This may be due to inexperience with the technique.

Endoscopic Lymph Node Biopsy

During this procedure, known as an *endoscopic lymph node biopsy* an endoscope is passed through the mouth and into the esophagus. An endoscope is a flexible device with a light attached that is used to look inside a body cavity or organ. After the scope is in the correct position, a biopsy tool may be used to sample nearby lymph nodes. No incision is required, and the patient does not require a general anesthetic.

Endobronchial Ultrasound

An *endobronchial ultrasound (EBUS)* is a procedure physicians commonly use to obtain biopsies of lymph nodes along the outside of the bronchial tree—the airways and their branches contained within the lungs. After an endoscope is in place down the throat, a physician uses a special probe to send ultrasound waves through the walls of the airways and into surrounding areas. If the physician sees abnormal lymph nodes, he or she can take a biopsy of them with a special needle.

Video-Assisted Thoracoscopy

A minimally invasive surgical technique, a *video-assisted thoracoscopy (VATS)* may be used to biopsy lung tumors. This procedure involves making a small incision in the chest and inserting a tiny video camera through a scope. The surgeon is then able to see the inside of the patient's chest on a television monitor. The biopsy is performed using surgical instruments that are placed through two or three other small incisions in the chest.

Exploratory Surgery

There are times when exploratory surgery must be performed to determine whether a lung tumor is a cancer. This may be the case if previous attempts to diagnose a tumor with less invasive tests have not produced conclusive results and if doctors are highly suspicious that a tumor is a cancer. During exploratory surgery, the tumor is removed. If the medical team discovers that the tumor is indeed malignant, then a complete

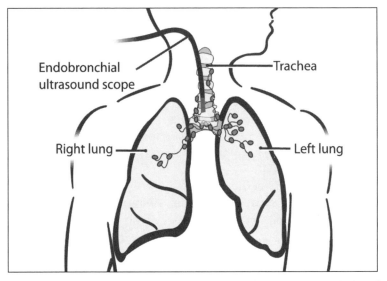

An endobronchial ultrasound (EBUS) is used to check for cancer cells in the lymph nodes in the center of the chest. A physician inserts a special scope through the trachea to obtain tissue samples.

cancer operation, such as removing a lobe of the lung and any affected lymph nodes, may be performed during the procedure.

Screening for Lung Cancer

Screening for a disease involves looking for it at an early stage before it causes any symptoms. As mentioned previously, treatment of lung cancer at an early stage improves the prospects of a cure. So should those at higher risk for lung cancer, such as smokers, be screened for the disease? The answer is yes, according to a study called the National Lung Screening Trial (NLST).

Sponsored by the National Cancer Institute, the NLST tracked fifty-three thousand people who smoked either a pack of cigarettes a day for thirty years or two packs a day for fifteen years. The study showed that when current and former heavy smokers got annual CT scans, they reduced their risk of death from lung cancer by 20 percent. The study also proved that the CT scan is more effective than a standard chest X-ray in detecting lung cancer, especially if the cancer is at an early stage.

Many physicians have accepted the CT scan as a valid screening test for lung cancer. The test, which takes only a few minutes, is available at most hospitals. However, CT scans can detect other abnormalities, such as nodules, which may or may not be cancerous. Therefore, additional tests may be necessary to determine whether a growth is malignant.

After the Diagnosis

If, after your medical tests, you are diagnosed with lung cancer, the next step involves determining the stage of your cancer. This staging process helps doctors determine the best course of treatment. In the chapter ahead, you'll learn how cancer is staged.

4 Staging Lung Cancer

The process of *staging* a newly discovered lung cancer involves determining the extent of the cancer's growth. For example, is the cancer at an early stage, meaning it has not spread beyond the lungs? Or, has the cancer spread outside the lungs, indicating that it is at a more advanced stage? Knowing the stage of a cancer is important because it helps doctors determine the best treatment path to follow.

Before your doctor can fully stage your lung cancer, he or she needs to answer the following questions:

- What is the size of the tumor?
- What is the extent of tumor growth?
- Are the lymph nodes near the tumor involved?
- Has the cancer spread to other organs?

Types of Staging

There are two types of staging: clinical and pathological. Clinical staging is based on your doctor's clinical findings—from the physical examination and any diagnostic tests, including X-rays, scans, and biopsies—prior to any form of treatment. Pathological staging is based on the clinical findings along with an analysis of tumor samples after surgery to remove the cancer if surgery has been performed.

If surgery is not performed, the staging of the disease is based on imaging scans, such as computerized tomography (CT), magnetic resonance imaging (MRI), and positron emission tomography (PET), after the cancer diagnosis is confirmed by biopsy.

The Pathology Report

After surgery to remove cancer, a pathologist will examine the tissues removed. He or she will measure the tumor and look at samples of the tumor and surrounding lung tissues through a microscope to determine the extent of the cancer. The pathologist will also look at any lymph nodes removed by the surgeon, to see if cancer cells are present.

When testing of the tissue specimens is complete, the pathologist will deliver a written pathology report to your doctor. (It usually takes several days after surgery to receive a final pathology report.) This report will tell your doctor the size of the cancer, the type of lung cancer, whether the cancer has spread beyond the lungs, and whether the lymph nodes are involved. The pathology report will help your doctor determine the stage of your cancer.

Size of the Cancer

The size of the tumor is the first factor to be considered in determining the stage of lung cancer. To determine the size, the pathologist typically uses a simple ruler to measure the largest part of the tumor.

Type of Cancer Cells Present

The pathologist will study the abnormal tissues to determine the type of cancer cells present. As noted in chapter 1, lung cancer is generally divided into two types: non-small cell and small cell. The non-small cell type is further identified as being either adenocarcinoma or squamous cell carcinoma.

Degree of Differentiation

Degree of differentiation refers to how much the cancer cells resemble normal cells. There are three degrees of differentiation: poorly, moderately, and well-differentiated. Within a given stage of cancer, tumors with poorly differentiated cells tend to be more aggressive than the other two types and signal the worst prognosis. Well-differentiated cancer cells tend to be not as aggressive and indicate the best prognosis.

Sites to which Lung Cancer Can Spread

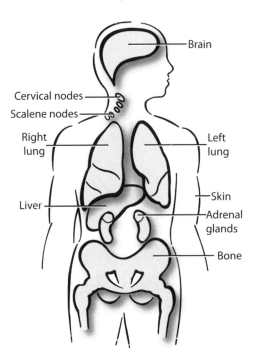

Spread to the Blood or Lymphatic Vessels

If cancer cells have invaded the walls of the blood or lymphatic vessels surrounding the tumor, they have the potential to spread to distant sites in the body via the bloodstream. This is not a favorable characteristic, because it increases the risk of the spread of cancer to other organs in the body.

Resection Margins

The term *resection* refers to the surgical removal of a cancer. *Resection margins* refer to the tissues at the edges of the tissue that a surgeon has removed. The pathologist will analyze these edge tissues for evidence of cancer cells. If the resection margins are free of cancer cells, it's an indication that all of the cancerous tissue was removed during the surgery. However, if the resection margins contain cancer cells, further treatment will be required.

Extent of Tumor Growth

This part of the pathology report describes how far the cancer has progressed. The best-case scenario is that the tumor is confined to the lung. A less favorable scenario is that the tumor has grown beyond the lung. A critical feature is whether the cancer has invaded the lining around the lung, called the *visceral pleura.* The farther the cancer has grown beyond the lung, the greater the chance of it spreading to the lymph nodes or to distant organs. The chances are also higher for *recurrence* of the cancer.

Lymph Node Involvement

The pathology report will tell whether the cancer has invaded lymph nodes. If the lymph nodes are reported to be "negative," it means no cancerous cells were found in them. A report of "positive" lymph nodes means cancer cells are present and further treatment will be needed. In addition, the number of lymph nodes involved is a factor in determining prognosis.

Stages of Non-Small Cell Lung Cancer

Taking into consideration all the information from the pathology report, your doctor will classify the stage of your lung cancer. For non-small cell lung cancer, the stages range from I to IV, with stage I being an early-stage cancer and stage IV being a late-stage cancer.

- *Stage I:* This is the earliest stage of non-small cell lung cancer. The cancer is found in only one lung and has not spread to any lymph nodes. Stage I is divided into two groups—stage IA, which is for smaller tumors, and stage IB, which is for larger tumors.
- *Stage II:* The cancer has spread to the lymph nodes that are contained within the surrounding affected lung.
- *Stage IIIA:* The cancer has spread to the lymph nodes

outside of the lung to those in the tracheal area, including the chest wall and the diaphragm on the side where the cancer started.

- *Stage IIIB:* The cancer has spread to the lymph nodes on the opposite lung or in the neck.
- *Stage IV:* The cancer has spread to other parts of the lungs or distantly throughout the body.

Note: For more details on the system that doctors use for classifying the extent to which a cancer has spread, see the "TNM Classification System" in the Appendix. You may wish to ask your physician to help you understand it.

Stages of Small Cell Lung Cancer

Small cell lung cancer is staged differently from non-small cell lung cancer. Small cell lung cancer is most commonly classified as either *limited stage* or *extensive stage*.

- *Limited stage:* The cancer is limited to the chest. It is found only in one lung and the nearby lymph nodes.
- *Extensive stage:* The cancer has spread beyond from the lung to other organs.

Treatment Based on the Stage of Cancer

As soon as the stage of your cancer is determined, your doctor can recommend the best type of treatment for you. For an early-stage non-small cell lung cancer, treatment may involve surgery alone. For other stages of this cancer and for small cell lung cancer, treatment plans may involve radiation or chemotherapy or a combination of both, with or without surgery.

Treatment Options by Stage
for Non-Small Cell Lung Cancer

- *Stage I:* Usually, surgery alone; radiation therapy alone in certain situations.
- *Stage II:* Surgery followed by chemotherapy.
- *Stage III:* Chemotherapy and radiation therapy

followed by surgery; chemotherapy and radiation without surgery; surgery followed by chemotherapy with or without radiation; chemotherapy followed by surgery.

- *Stage IV:* Usually chemotherapy alone; possible surgery for single sites to which cancer may have spread, such as the brain or adrenal glands.

Treatment Options by Stage for Small Cell Lung Cancer

- *Limited stage:* Chemotherapy and radiation therapy; sometimes surgery.
- *Extensive stage:* Chemotherapy, clinical trials, and supportive care.

Multimodality Treatment

Today, the optimal treatment for lung cancer is a *multimodality approach.* This means delivering multiple types of treatment—surgery, radiation therapy, and chemotherapy—rather than a single form of treatment. Research has shown that tailored multimodality treatment regimens simplify the treatment process and produce better patient outcomes.

Multimodality therapy is best administered by a health care team that confers regularly on a given case. All members of this team of physicians and other health care professionals take part in all the steps related to care: diagnosis, staging, treatment, and even long-term follow-up.

In the chapters ahead, you'll learn about the treatment options—surgery, radiation therapy, and chemotherapy.

5 Surgery

Whether or not you are a candidate for surgery depends on the type of lung cancer you have, whether it has spread beyond the lung, and how well your lungs function. Between 10 and 35 percent of lung cancer patients are candidates for surgery.

The goal of surgery in treating lung cancer is to cure the patient—to remove all cancer. Removing only a portion of the cancer would not improve the patient's chance of survival and, thus, would unnecessarily expose him or her to risks related to the surgery. Therefore, surgery is recommended only when it seems very likely that the surgeon can remove all cancer and the patient is strong enough to undergo surgery.

With modern imaging studies such as computerized tomography (CT) and positron emission tomography (PET) scans, doctors can more accurately estimate whether all visible cancer can be removed with surgery. Even so, in some instances, a surgeon's determination of whether the cancer can be completely removed can only be made after he or she has looked into the chest cavity during surgery.

Preparing for Lung Cancer Surgery

Before performing an operation to remove part or all of a person's lung, a surgeon makes certain that the amount of lung remaining after the operation will be sufficient to allow the patient to live without being incapacitated. Your surgeon may refer you to a *pulmonologist*, a physician who specializes in

Pneumonectomy

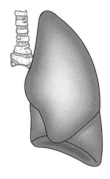

Lobectomy

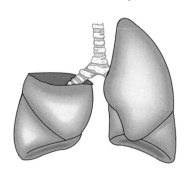

medical treatment for the lungs. The pulmonologist will likely have you undergo *pulmonary function tests.* These tests evaluate lung function by measuring the amount of air you breathe in and out. A diffusing capacity test measures how well the tiny blood vessels in the lungs function. Sometimes, a perfusion scan is performed to measure the amount of blood flowing to one lung compared to the other lung.

Types of Lung Cancer Surgery

Lung cancer surgery may be performed by a general surgeon or a thoracic surgeon, a surgeon who specializes in surgery for the chest and lungs. If it is determined that your treatment should include surgery, the surgeon will choose from several types of surgical procedures for lung cancer. The type of procedure performed depends on the size and location of the tumor.

Pneumonectomy: This procedure involves the removal of an entire lung.

Lobectomy: The most commonly performed surgery for lung cancer, a lobectomy is the removal of a lobe containing cancer.

Sleeve lobectomy: This procedure involves the removal of a lobe and a portion of the air passage tube (bronchus) to which it is attached. Then, the remaining part of the bronchus is attached to a remaining lobe.

Wedge resection: With this procedure, a wedge of lung tissue containing cancer is removed. Wedge resections typically are used to remove small lung tumors.

Segmentectomy: The surgical removal of a segment is called a segmentectomy. (The lobes of the lungs are made up of segments.) This procedure is used to remove small tumors.

Lymphadenectomy: In addition to removing the tumor, the surgeon must also remove lymph nodes from within the affected lung, along with lymph nodes in the mediastinum, the area in the chest between the lungs. The removal of lymph nodes is called a *lymphadenectomy*. A pathologist will examine the lymph nodes to determine whether they contain cancer. As mentioned earlier, doctors must know the stage of a cancer in order to determine the best treatment plan. Furthermore, patients who do not have

Sleeve lobectomy

Removed segment of bronchus

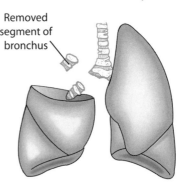

Wedge resection

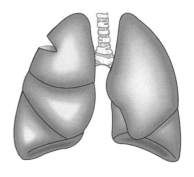

Segmentectomy

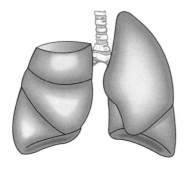

their lymph nodes sampled may not be eligible for certain clinical trials or state-of-the-art cancer therapies.

An operation for lung cancer is not complete if mediastinal lymph node samples are not taken and then sent to a pathologist. Ask your surgeon if he or she plans to sample the mediastinal lymph nodes during the surgery; if the answer is no, seek a second opinion.

Surgical Techniques

Thoracotomy

A *thoracotomy* is a surgical procedure that involves cutting through the chest wall to gain access to the chest cavity. It is the most commonly used procedure for removing part or all of a lung.

For a thoracotomy, the patient receives general anesthesia and is completely asleep. An anesthesiologist inserts breathing tubes into each lung; air flow to the lung being operated on is stopped and the lung deflated. This makes it easier for the surgeon to operate. Then, the surgeon makes a five- to ten-inch incision that starts under the shoulder blade and extends around to the back. The surgeon carefully divides the underlying muscles and spreads the ribs apart to gain access to the lung. Sometimes, the surgeon will remove a small piece of rib bone in order to better see inside the chest.

When the operation is complete, the lung is reinflated if it has not been totally removed and the surgeon closes the incision with sutures. The patient may spend the first day or two after surgery in the intensive care unit where hospital staff can carefully monitor him or her. The typical hospital stay after a thoracotomy is four to six days.

Minimally Invasive Procedures

Minimally invasive surgery is increasingly being used by surgeons to operate on the lungs. Instead of making a large incision and spreading the ribs to gain access to the chest cavity, the surgeon makes two or three small (one inch or less) incisions between the ribs. This approach may be used to perform lobectomies, segmentectomies, and wedge resections.

Minimally invasive procedures are associated with less pain and a faster recovery. The two main types of minimally invasive procedures are *video-assisted thoracic surgery* and *robotic-assisted thoracic surgery*.

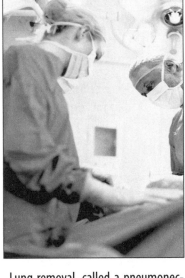

Lung removal, called a pneumonectomy, is a major surgery that requires a stay of several days in the hospital.

As described in chapter 3, video-assisted thoracic surgery (VATS) involves a surgeon operating by inserting surgical instruments through small incisions in the chest; the surgeon first passes a tube, containing a tiny television camera, into the chest. The procedure is used to perform biopsies, but it can also be used to perform what's called an *excisional biopsy* in which an entire tumor is removed. This procedure can also be used to remove a lobe of a lung.

To undergo this procedure, the patient must receive a general anesthetic. Video-assisted thoracic surgery has become a commonly accepted method for treating early-stage lung cancer (stages I and II).

Robotic-assisted thoracic surgery uses the same small incisions as the video-assisted technique, but the operation is performed using a special instrument with a robotic arm to manipulate the lung tissue within the chest.

Recovering in the Hospital

Removing part or all of a lung is a major operation. Patients usually spend at least a few days to a week recovering in the hospital. Sometimes, patients will spend the first day or two after surgery in an intensive care unit.

Potential Complications

Most patients recover from their surgery and go home within a few days. However, complications are possible. These include pneumonia, wound infection, blood clots, bleeding, and irregular heartbeat (palpitations). These complications can prolong recovery and the length of the hospital stay. However, your health care team will assist you and encourage you to take certain actions to help prevent complications from occurring after surgery.

Chest Tube for Drainage

After surgery, you'll have a drainage tube coming out of your chest. The lungs are normally lubricated with fluid, but the amount of fluid can increase from inflammation caused by the surgery. The chest tube drains this fluid and also allows for leaking air to escape. After surgery, it's normal for air to leak through any tiny holes in the thin tissue that covers the lung; such holes usually heal and seal themselves after a few days. Until then, the chest tube prevents pressure from the leaking air from building up.

The chest tube may be left in place for several days after your surgery. It is usually removed when there is no longer any drainage or leaking air.

Preventing Pneumonia

Pneumonia is the most common complication after lung surgery. Breathing deeply helps keep the lungs expanded, which helps prevent pneumonia. Taking deep breaths at least every hour while awake is the most important measure you can take to prevent pneumonia after lung surgery.

Concentrate on your breathing while recovering in the hospital. An *incentive spirometer* can help you keep your lungs expanded. This is a tube-like device that you inhale through. It has a gauge that shows how well your lungs expand.

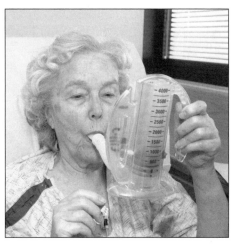

Using an incentive spirometer to take deep breaths helps keep the lungs expanded after surgery. *Photo by CMSP*

Begin Light Exercise

Getting out of bed and beginning light, supervised exercise is important to your recovery in the hospital. Taking short walks three to four times a day is the most important thing you can do to prevent blood clots and speed your recovery after surgery. When you stand up to walk, you give your lungs more room to expand, preventing pneumonia. When you use your leg muscles, blood is pumped up from the veins in your legs, which helps prevent blood clots from forming. Walking also helps prevent postoperative constipation, which can lead to bloating that, in turn, can make it harder to take deep breaths. Also, when you walk, your body uses insulin more effectively, helping to control your blood sugar.

Managing Pain

While you're still in the hospital, your health care team will work to manage postsurgical pain. If your pain is managed, you'll recover more quickly.

In addition to pain pills, many hospitals use *patient-controlled anesthesia (PCA)*, which allows the patient to push a button and receive pain medication through an *intravenous (IV) line*. Another method of pain control is a *thoracic epidural catheter.* With this method, an anesthesiologist inserts a thin tube into your back. Pain medication is delivered through the tube and the chest area is numbed.

Recovering at Home

Recovering at home after lung cancer surgery can take several weeks. During this time, watch for any signs of infection—fever, drainage, redness, increasing pain from your incision, or coughing up dark sputum. If you notice any of these warning signs of infection, contact your surgeon immediately.

Continue Pain Control

You may require pain management for as long as a week or two after you return home from the hospital. Your doctor will give you a prescription for pain medication to take at home. Remember, the best way to manage pain is to take the medication *before* the pain worsens. In other words, don't "chase" the pain—stay ahead of it.

Unfortunately, some patients don't use their pain medication as often as they should, fearing that they are not being "good" patients or that they may become addicted to the medication. Neither of these concerns is valid. You're not being a "bad" patient by using pain pills; in fact, keeping your pain under control will help you heal faster. And using pain medication as directed to treat postsurgical pain does not cause addiction.

Regain Strength Gradually

Do not expect to have a normal energy level right away. It will take one to two months for your energy to return to its preoperative level. Do not try to do too much too fast. Limit your activities, and do not expect to return to work for at least one month. While you are recovering, expect your energy level to fluctuate, alternating between good days and bad days. This is normal after major surgery.

Manage Emotions

In addition to being a physical strain, recovering at home from lung cancer surgery can be full of emotional ups and downs. This kind of mental stress is especially common when you are at home and inactive. Many people find it helpful to keep busy at home with hobbies and activities that exercise their mental capabilities.

Do not be afraid to open up to trusted family members and friends. Talk with them about how you're feeling, your fears, and your concerns. Some people find comfort in support groups, which can provide both moral support and practical advice for recovery. Some individuals find it helpful to speak with a clergy person or a professional counselor.

Follow-up after Surgery

After your discharge from the hospital, you'll be scheduled for a series of follow-up appointments with your surgeon. It's common to see your surgeon at least every six months for the first two to three years. These medical checkups typically include a physical examination, a CT scan, and blood testing. The intention is to detect any cancer recurrence early so that it can be treated immediately. These appointments are also an opportunity for you to tell your surgeon about any problems or symptoms you're having.

6 Radiation Therapy

Approximately 50 percent of lung cancer patients undergo radiation therapy as part of their treatment. Basically, radiation therapy is similar to X-rays. However, unlike X-rays, radiation therapy kills cancer cells by delivering carefully targeted beams of high-intensity radiation into cancerous tissues. The radiation is delivered with the help of sophisticated scanning equipment, such as computerized tomography (CT) scanners, that enable oncologists to see tumors.

A *radiation oncologist* is a physician who specializes in treating cancer with radiation therapy. This physician will discuss with you the type of lung cancer you have, its stage, and your overall health to determine whether radiation therapy should be part of your treatment plan.

How Radiation Therapy Works

Radiation kills cells that multiply rapidly. Because cancer cells multiply in a rapid, chaotic fashion, radiation can stop them from reproducing. Healthy cells may also be affected by radiation, but they are not as vulnerable to it as are fast-growing cancer cells. The goal of radiation therapy is to eliminate cancer cells and spare the surrounding healthy cells; however, some damage to healthy cells is often unavoidable. Fortunately, normal cells are able to repair themselves over time.

The most commonly used radiation treatment for lung cancer is *external beam radiation therapy*, or *EBRT*. This type of treatment sends radiation rays into a tumor from outside the body. EBRT may be used to treat a tumor in the lung or tumors in other organs to which cancer may have spread.

Several health care professionals are involved in the delivery of radiation therapy. In addition to a radiation oncologist, they include a *medical radiation physicist*, who makes sure that the radiation is properly tailored to the patient; a *medical dosimetrist*, who calculates the dosages; and a *radiation therapist*, who delivers the actual treatments.

Combining Radiation Therapy with Other Treatments

Radiation therapy may be given alone, as a primary treatment for lung cancer, or it may be used in combination with other treatments. For example, if you are scheduled for surgery, you may have radiation therapy before the surgery to shrink the tumor so that the surgeon has a better chance of removing the entire tumor. When radiation is given prior to surgery, it is called *neoadjuvant therapy*.

Radiation therapy may also be used after surgery. In this case, it is used with the intention of killing any cancer cells that may remain in the body after surgery. Radiation therapy given after surgery is called *adjuvant therapy*. After surgery, radiation may also be used to treat other organs to which cancer may have spread.

Radiation therapy is also often prescribed to treat lung cancer when surgery isn't an option. It may also be used for *palliative treatment*—that is, to relieve symptoms such as shortness of breath, bleeding, trouble swallowing, cough, discomfort, and pain—when the cancer has progressed.

Radiation therapy may be used in combination with chemotherapy before or after surgery. It may also be combined with chemotherapy when surgery is not part of the treatment plan.

Before Your First Treatment

Before your first radiation treatment, you will have a *simulation appointment*. This is essentially a treatment planning session during which your radiation team will determine

37

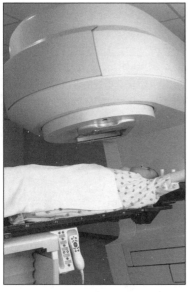

External beam radiation is delivered through a linear accelerator. Treatment for lung cancer is commonly given five days a week for several weeks.

the precise area to be treated. This planning ensures that the radiation beam will be aimed accurately during each treatment. Part of this planning involves determining the best position for your body during treatment and the angles at which the beams will enter your body.

During the simulation, you'll be asked to lie in the same position that you'll lie in for your treatments. Most likely, you will be on your back or abdomen. You may be fitted with an immobilization device. This device is a comfortable, yet rigid, cradle that holds your body in place during each treatment. It is created by pouring resin or polystyrene beads into a bag made of urethane, nylon, or another sturdy material. The bag is then molded to the specific contours of your body.

During the simulation, you may receive an injection of contrast material, followed by a CT scan or another imaging scan. The contrast material is a liquid that travels through the body and improves the visibility of both the internal structures and the tumor itself. Then, the radiation therapy staff will take measurements, enabling them to pinpoint the area to be treated.

After the treatment area is determined, a radiation therapist will make tiny dots on your skin, which will indicate the area where the radiation beam will be aimed. These tiny dots may be made with a marker or a tattoo, either of which must stay in place throughout your therapy. If the tiny marks are tattooed on your skin, they can be removed later with a laser or simply left in place. Since they're tiny, like freckles, patients rarely find them bothersome after treatment.

Receiving Radiation Treatments

During an actual treatment, you'll lie on a table while a machine called a *linear accelerator* moves in various directions around your body, sending radiation beams into the tumor. This machine is programmed to deliver precisely calculated dosages of radiation, referred to as high-energy X-rays. Each treatment lasts only a few minutes.

Radiation therapy for lung cancer is usually given five days a week, over three to seven weeks. It's given over a period of time because higher dosages over a shorter period of time would be too destructive to healthy cells and would create more serious side effects. With the treatments spread over a longer period of time, the cancer cells can still be attacked while minimizing damage to healthy cells.

Types of Radiation Therapy

Three-Dimensional Conformal Radiation Therapy

One form of external beam radiation therapy, *three-dimensional conformal radiation therapy (3D-CRT)*, offers precision in treating a tumor because the radiation beams actually conform to, or match, the shape of the tumor. This technique reduces the likelihood of damage to healthy tissues. Physicians use special CT scanners and computers to precisely map the tumor's outline in three dimensions. Then the radiation beams, shaped to match the shape of the tumor, are delivered from multiple angles.

Intensity Modulated Radiation Therapy

Another specialized form of radiation therapy, *intensity modulated radiation therapy (IMRT)*, takes three-dimensional conformal radiation therapy one step further. Beyond shaping the radiation beams to precisely outline the tumor, IMRT allows radiation oncologists to break up the radiation beams into smaller "beamlets" and adjust their intensity. Physicians can deliver even higher dosages of radiation while minimizing damage to nearby healthy tissues. This form of radiation therapy is especially useful in treating lung tumors near the heart or spinal cord.

Image-Guided Radiation Therapy

Image-guided radiation therapy (IGRT) is yet another advanced form of radiation treatment. With this technique, doctors are able to use CT scans to monitor the organ being treated during the treatment. This is valuable in treating lung cancer because a tumor can change position as a patient breathes. During IGRT, the doctor can compare the CT scans with earlier scans and make any needed adjustments in tailoring the focus of radiation beams.

Stereotactic Radiation Therapy

Stereotactic radiation therapy (SRT) is a specialized form of external beam radiation therapy that delivers multiple beams of radiation in high dosages. It is often recommended for people with early-stage lung cancer who are not candidates for surgery. When planning the treatment, doctors map out both the tumor's shape and the lung's motion. Tiny markers are placed into the lung to assist in accurately targeting the tumor. The insertion of these markers is performed during a procedure much like a biopsy.

During a treatment, several high dosages of radiation are delivered, as opposed to many small dosages. Because the radiation beam is tightly focused, healthy tissues are not as susceptible to injury, and the chances of side effects occurring are minimized. Treatment time is also shorter. One to five treatments are administered over a two-week period, compared to daily treatments over several weeks for conventional radiation.

Brachytherapy

Unlike radiation therapy that uses external beams of radiation, *brachytherapy*, also called *internal radiation therapy*, attacks cancer cells from inside the body. This therapy involves the placement of radioactive "seeds" directly into a tumor or near it. Brachytherapy is commonly used to relieve symptoms such as bleeding or to open blocked airways.

To deliver brachytherapy, a physician performs a bronchoscopy, which involves the insertion of a flexible, lighted tube through the mouth and into the lungs to examine the airways and lungs. The physician then inserts thin, hollow plastic catheters into the airways through a nostril. The radioactive seeds are delivered through the catheters to the tumor site. However, since this form of therapy involves high-dosage radiation, the seeds are then removed immediately. Several treatments are required. Each treatment takes from thirty-five to fifty minutes.

Brachytherapy also can be performed by inserting lower-dosage seeds at the time of surgery. The seeds stay in place permanently after treatment. These seeds remain active for a period of time, eventually becoming inactive and harmless to the body.

Side Effects of Radiation Therapy

Radiation treatments themselves are not painful; however, the treatments do produce side effects. Some of the side effects can be uncomfortable and distressing; however, they're usually temporary and treatable. They're also unique to each patient—not every patient will have the same side effects.

Fatigue

Many patients report feeling tired during radiation therapy. The fatigue may increase as the treatments continue; however, usually it only becomes severe if a patient is receiving chemotherapy at the same time or is very ill. When fatigue is caused only by the radiation therapy, it usually eases over the ensuing weeks and months after completion of the therapy. Until then, you can counter any fatigue by following these tips:

- Stay as active as possible; mild exercise, such as a brisk, 20-minute walk each day, can help reenergize you.
- Get plenty of rest.
- Work within your tolerance, taking time off if necessary.

- Eat a healthy diet with enough protein and calories to keep both your weight and your energy up.
- Drink six to eight glasses of water daily to stay hydrated and energized.

Hair Loss

If you're a man, you're likely to lose chest hair in areas penetrated by the radiation beams. This hair loss may be temporary or permanent, depending on how much radiation is delivered.

If radiation therapy is directed at your brain, in the event of the cancer spreading to the brain, you'll lose the hair on your head. In many cases, the hair grows back, depending on the amount of scalp hair in the treatment area and on the dosage of the radiation. However, hair may grow back in a slightly different color, texture, or density.

Skin Irritation

Skin irritation is one of the most common side effects of radiation therapy. As treatment progresses over a few weeks, any chest skin in the path of the radiation beams can become red, dry, tender, or itchy. It can even peel like sunburn. In most cases, the skin returns to normal after therapy; however, in some cases, it may be permanently rough and darkened. During therapy, you can diminish skin irritation by taking these steps:

- Wear loose-fitting clothes.
- Clean your skin with lukewarm water; avoid hot water and soaps when bathing.
- Pat your skin dry rather than rub it; don't scratch your skin, either.
- Keep the treatment area out of direct sunlight; use sunscreen when necessary.
- Refrain from using heating pads or ice packs on the treatment area.
- Refrain from using any perfumes or perfumed products, including powders, cosmetics, and deodorants; ask your doctor for advice on unscented creams or lotions.

Dry, Sore Throat or Cough

Radiation therapy can cause temporary irritation of the airways if the treatment field includes your throat. The irritation can lead to a scratchy or sore throat and an accompanying cough. You can address these problems as follows:

- Moisturize the air in your home or workplace with a humidifier or vaporizer.
- Stay out of smoke-filled environments; refrain from smoking cigarettes, cigars, or pipes and from chewing tobacco.
- Suck on sugarless mints to increase your production of saliva.
- Drink enough liquids to keep your mucus thin.
- Gargle with warm saltwater (one-half teaspoon of salt mixed with eight ounces of water).

Be sure to ask your doctor before using any over-the-counter cough medicines, mouthwashes, or lozenges. If necessary, your radiation oncologist will prescribe medication.

Painful Swallowing

Inability to swallow without discomfort is common with radiation therapy if the radiation beams are aimed near the *esophagus*, the tube that carries food from the mouth to the stomach. The resulting inflammation, called *esophagitis*, can be severe, especially if you're undergoing chemotherapy at the same time. Esophagitis makes swallowing painful and difficult to the point that you may not want to eat, which can result in weight loss. The inflammation should disappear within several weeks of completing therapy. However, during therapy, you can minimize the discomfort by following these tips:

- Eat a soft or pureed diet with no temperature extremes.
- Avoid foods that are spicy or acidic.
- Cut food in small pieces, and eat the pieces with broth, gravy, or sauces added.
- Eat smaller meals more often during the day to keep your energy up and ease digestion.

- Drink at least four to six glasses of liquid each day, but refrain from coffee, tea, other caffeinated drinks, and alcohol.

Your radiation oncologist can prescribe medications if you need it.

Radiation Pneumonitis

Between 5 and 15 percent of lung cancer patients undergoing radiation therapy experience *radiation pneumonitis*, an inflammation of the lungs. The risk for this condition depends on the radiation dosage and the size of the area treated. Radiation pneumonitis can cause chest pain, coughing, fever, and sometimes shortness of breath. It usually gets better within several weeks with no treatment. Your doctor, however, may prescribe steroids, such as prednisone, as well as antibiotics and/or cough suppressants to ease the symptoms.

Pulmonary Fibrosis

A long-term side effect that may occur from radiation theapy is the development of scar tissue in the area of the lung that was treated. This scarring, called *pulmonary fibrosis*, may occur months to years after treatment. Symptoms of pulmonary fibrosis include shortness of breath, dry cough, and chest pain. Treatment may include steroids, use of oxygen, and pulmonary rehabilitation to increase lung efficiency.

After Radiation Therapy

After you have completed your radiation therapy, your radiation oncologist will want to examine you within a few weeks for any side effects. It's not uncommon to develop radiation pneumonitis within a few months after you've completed treatment. As mentioned, most individuals have a complete recovery from this condition.

Your radiation oncologist will want to do additional examinations in the months ahead. These follow-up checkups will include a physical examination, X-rays, and imaging scans.

7 Chemotherapy

Chemotherapy plays a major role in cancer treatment. It is used to help cure, control, or ease the symptoms of cancer. Nearly half of all cancer patients undergo chemotherapy.

If your doctor decides that chemotherapy is right for you, you'll meet with a *medical oncologist*, a doctor who specializes in chemotherapy. He or she will formulate a chemotherapy plan to treat your cancer.

How Chemotherapy Works

Most chemotherapy agents work by killing rapidly dividing cells. Cancer cells are rapidly dividing cells. Some normal cells, such as those in the hair follicles and the lining of the mouth, are also rapidly dividing cells, and they, too, are affected by chemotherapy; however, normal cells are capable of recovering.

A newer class of chemotherapy drugs, called *targeted therapies*, do not work by attacking all fast-growing cells. Instead, they target structures within the cancer cells themselves. Some targeted therapies attack molecules within the cancer cells to keep the cells from reproducing. Other targeted therapies inhibit cancer growth by attacking cells on the surface of a tumor. Still other targeted therapies target the blood vessels that supply oxygen to a tumor.

Chemotherapy after Surgery

Chemotherapy is given after lung cancer surgery with the intention of killing any cancer cells that might have already

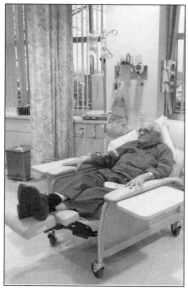

Intravenous chemotherapy treatments, called infusions, are usually given at an out-patient center. *Photo by CMSP*

escaped into the bloodstream before the surgery. It's not possible for doctors to know when microscopic cancer cells have entered the bloodstream; however, if they consider a person at high risk for this based on the stage of his or her cancer (stage II or higher), they will recommend chemotherapy. Other factors that determine whether chemotherapy is appropriate after surgery include the type of lung cancer, how aggressive it is, the patient's age, and the overall health of the patient. When chemotherapy is given after surgery, it is called *adjuvant chemotherapy.*

If you've undergone surgery, your physician will probably wait three to four weeks before beginning chemotherapy to allow you time to heal from the surgery. The schedules for chemotherapy vary depending on the type of chemotherapy agent being used. Typically, a treatment would be given every three weeks. For example, a schedule could involve receiving a total of six treatments—one treatment every three weeks over a four- to five-month period.

After your chemotherapy treatments have begun, your oncologist will do periodic evaluations at to determine your response to the chemotherapy. If you are responding well, you may be switched to a maintenance dosage of chemotherapy. In this case, you will receive a treatment once every week or every three weeks, depending on the type of agent being used. This will likely continue for several months.

If your oncologist determines that you are not responding to the chemotherapy, he or she will likely switch you to a different type of chemotherapy agent and reevaluate your response at three and six months. Typically, treatments will be given every three weeks.

Chemotherapy before Surgery

A doctor may recommend chemotherapy before surgery for lung cancer that may have spread locally to lymph nodes in the center of the chest. The goal here is to eliminate as many cancer cells as possible in order to increase the surgeon's chances of successfully removing all the cancer. Chemotherapy prior to surgery is called *neoadjuvant chemotherapy.*

Chemotherapy before lung cancer surgery usually lasts four months, with surgery following three to four weeks after completion of the chemotherapy. In some cases, radiation therapy may be given along with the chemotherapy.

Palliative Chemotherapy

Another form of treatment, palliative chemotherapy, is often given to provide relief from symptoms. Palliative chemotherapy may be an option when cancer has already spread to other organs at the time of initial diagnosis. In such cases, chemotherapy may shrink a tumor and slow its growth.

Chemotherapy Treatments

The medications used for chemotherapy treatments consist of a group of different drugs. These medications may be used individually or in combination with each other.

Chemotherapy treatments are given in cycles. You receive a treatment followed by a recovery period. Then you have another treatment followed by another recovery period. Why are treatments given in cycles? As explained earlier, chemotherapy kills the cancer cells that are rapidly dividing—but it won't affect cancer cells that are at rest. Giving the treatments in cycles intensifies the effort to kill cancer cells when they are in the reproduction phase. The time off between treatments also helps normal tissues recover.

> **Chemotherapy Agents and Targeted Therapy Drugs**
> *Generic Names and Trade Names*
>
> **Chemotherapy Agents**
>
> - Cisplatin (*Platinol*)
> - Carboplatin (*Paraplatin*)
> - Paclitaxel (*Taxol, Onxol*)
> - Docetaxel (*Taxotare*)
> - Gemcitabine (*Gemzar*)
> - Vinorelbine (*Navelbine*)
> - Irinotecan (*Camptosar, Camptothecin-11*)
> - Etoposide (*Toposar, VePesid, Etopophos*)
> - Vinblastine (*Velban, Alkaban-AQ*)
> - Pemetrexed (*Alimta*)
>
> **Targeted Therapy Drugs**
>
> - Becacizubab (*Avastin*)
> - Erlotinib (*Tarceva*)
> - Crizotinib (*Xalkori*)

Most chemotherapy treatments are given intravenously—the treatments are called infusions. Indeed, pills would be easier, but stomach acids and enzymes would break down some medications and prevent them from working. However, there are some chemotherapy drugs that are given in pill form.

Treatments are given in an outpatient setting, usually in a hospital's infusion center. A nurse who specializes in giving chemotherapy treatments will connect the intravenous (IV) line that delivers the chemotherapy. Before the treatment begins, the patient will be given anti-nausea medication. Nurses will monitor the patient carefully during the treatment.

While you're receiving an infusion, you'll be seated in a comfortable reclining chair. The treatment may last from one and one-half hours to four hours, depending on the chemotherapy agent used. During this time, you'll be able to read, watch television, use a laptop computer, or have visitors.

Chemotherapy through a Port

Chemotherapy for lung cancer is given over an extended period of time. So, to make the treatment process more efficient and more comfortable for you, your doctor will want to avoid your receiving a new IV line in your arm during each treatment. Accordingly, your chemotherapy may be delivered through a *port*.

A port is a small reservoir, about the size of a quarter, typically made of soft plastic. This port is surgically implanted in your chest just under the skin, usually under the collarbone. A soft, thin tube runs from the port into a large vein. The implantation of the port is an outpatient procedure, performed by your surgeon, and takes thirty to sixty minutes. Local anesthesia is used, and you may be given a mild sedative.

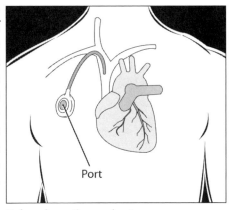

Before chemotherapy begins, a surgeon may implant a port, a small reservoir, under the skin. Chemotherapy infusions will be given through this port.

After the procedure, a chest X-ray is done to check the positioning of the port and to make sure there are no kinks in the tube. From this point, you'll receive your infusions through this port. Initially, when not in use, the port is covered with a bandage; once the small incision heals, no bandage is needed. The port requires no special care by the patient.

Ports rarely create complications; however, pain, redness, or swelling may indicate infection or clotting. You should report any such symptoms to your doctor immediately. Once you have completed your treatments, your surgeon will remove the port during an office visit.

Monitoring during Chemotherapy

You will be monitored closely while you're undergoing chemotherapy. Your blood count will be taken regularly to measure your red blood cells, platelets, and white blood cells. Your doctor will be watching for blood counts that drop too low. For example, if your white blood cell count drops, you'll be at risk for infections, because white blood cells fight infections.

In most people, blood counts drop to their lowest levels

seven to ten days after each treatment. This lowest point is called the *nadir*. When you are at your nadir, your immune system is weakened, and you will be particularly susceptible to infections. You may require medications that boost your white blood cell count during this period.

Can you continue working while undergoing chemotherapy? Many people do continue during the period they are undergoing treatments. Whether you can continue to work depends on your overall health and the nature of your job.

Side Effects of Chemotherapy

As mentioned previously, chemotherapy kills cancer cells that are rapidly reproducing. However, chemotherapy drugs will also attack normal, healthy cells that reproduce rapidly. As a result, side effects can occur.

The type of chemotherapy you receive, the dosage, and the duration of your treatment are factors in the types of side effects you may experience. It's important to note that not all patients experience every side effect, and when side effects do occur, they can usually be managed with prescription medications or even home remedies. Most side effects subside once the treatments end.

Fatigue

One of the most common side effects of chemotherapy for lung cancer is fatigue. Fatigue can be brought on by a low red blood cell count. Red blood cells deliver oxygen to the body, and if your red blood cell count is low, tissues and organs are not receiving adequate oxygen. As a result, you'll feel fatigued. This condition is called *anemia*. If you become severely anemic during chemotherapy, you may need a blood transfusion or medication that stimulates production of red blood cells.

For some patients, fatigue occurs around the time of a treatment. Others feel fatigued during the entire course of therapy. The fatigue may last even after chemotherapy has ended; it may take weeks for your energy level to return to normal. For normally active patients, the fatigue can be a source of frustration or even depression. Try to stay positive and remember that the fatigue is temporary. Here are a few tips for coping with fatigue:

- Limit your activities; do only those things that are most important to you.
- Take several short naps or breaks during the day.
- Try taking short walks or exercising lightly.
- Maintain good nutrition; try to eat a well-balanced diet.
- Ask for help when you need it.

Nausea and Vomiting

Nausea and vomiting are common side effects of chemotherapy used to treat lung cancer. However, if you experience these side effects, your oncologist can prescribe medications that will help. If vomiting persists for twenty-four hours, notify your doctor. You may need to be admitted to the hospital for intravenous fluids and medication. Here are other tips for managing nausea and vomiting:

- Take antinausea medications as directed.
- Breathe deeply and slowly when you feel nauseated.
- Drink six to eight glasses of water daily.
- Eat small, frequent meals rather than three large ones.
- Eat and drink slowly; chew foods well.
- Avoid rich, spicy foods.
- Suck on ice cubes, mints, or ginger candies (unless you have mouth sores).

Some people find that the smell of food cooking bothers them. If the smell of food makes your nausea worse, try staying out of the kitchen while food is being cooked.

Hair Loss

Chemotherapy can affect hair follicles, causing temporary hair loss. Although hair loss can occur anywhere on the body, it is mainly confined to the head. During chemotherapy, some people wear hats, scarves, or wigs to cover their heads and stay warm. To cope with hair loss, try these suggestions:

- Use mild shampoos.
- Use a soft hairbrush.
- Use low heat on your hair dryer.
- Don't use brush rollers to set your hair.
- Don't dye your hair or get a permanent.
- Have your hair cut short; a shorter style will make hair look thicker and fuller.
- Protect your scalp from the sun with a hat, a scarf, or sunscreen.

Once treatments are completed, hair grows back. It may grow back a slightly different color or texture.

Neuropathy

Chemotherapy can cause *neuropathy*, which is damage to nerve endings. When this occurs, you may have pain, numbness, or tingling sensations in various parts of the body. The severity of these side effects depends on the amount of the chemotherapy agent you received and how quickly it was administered. It's important to report these side effects to your oncologist right away so that he or she can adjust or suspend treatment before the side effects become severe.

Commonly, neuropathy occurs in the hands and feet; when it occurs in the hands, it may interfere with activities such as buttoning a shirt, typing, writing, or playing a musical instrument. Neuropathy can also occur in the mouth, throat, or chest; this may result in abnormal tongue sensations, a choking sensation, or a sensation of pressure on your chest.

Neuropathy may be either acute or chronic. Acute neuropathy goes away within days of a chemotherapy treatment, while chronic neuropathy can persist for weeks to months. Neuropathy symptoms may be constant, or they may come and go. The chronic form of neuropathy may become irreversible if treatment continues, so oncologists usually reduce the dosage of the chemotherapy agent or stop the treatment altogether. Medications are also available to alleviate neuropathy pain.

Infections

Chemotherapy can damage cells in the bone marrow, which is important in the production of infection-fighting white blood cells. As noted previously, when your white blood cell count is low, it may lead to a weakening of the immune system. This condition, known as neutropenia, makes you susceptible to infections, including pneumonia, blood infections, urine infections, and skin infections.

Be alert for the signs of infection—fever over 100 degrees Fahrenheit, shaking, chills, sweats, coughing up dark or bloody sputum, pain or burning with urination, and pain or redness around cuts. If you feel an infection coming on, notify your doctor immediately. Infections can be effectively treated with antibiotics.

To reduce your risk of infection, take these precautions:

- Wash your hands often during the day, especially after using the bathroom.
- Avoid anyone who has a cold, flu, measles, or chicken pox.
- Stay away from children who have recently received vaccinations.
- Clean cuts and scrapes right away.
- Wear gloves when gardening or cleaning up after pets or children.
- Use a soft toothbrush that won't hurt your gums.
- Clean your anus thoroughly after each bowel movement; if the area around your anus becomes irritated or if you have hemorrhoids, notify your doctor.

Impaired Blood Clotting

Chemotherapy can also cause a condition called *thrombocytopenia*, which means low blood platelet count. Platelets are the cells that help blood to clot. Mild cases of thrombocytopenia may produce no symptoms. However, if the platelet count drops low enough, symptoms may appear. One symptom is easy bruising, which means bleeding has occurred in the small blood vessels under the skin. Shallow bleeding in the skin can also cause a purplish rash on the hands and feet. Another symptom is spontaneous nosebleeds. In serious cases, internal bleeding may occur.

There are no medications for this condition, and a physician will usually delay or suspend chemotherapy treatment when a patient's blood platelet count is low. This break in treatment gives the platelet count time to increase on its own. If the platelet count drops dangerously low, however, a blood platelet transfusion may be needed to avoid bleeding complications.

Once the course of chemotherapy has ended, low blood counts are treatable and reversible. Throughout your treatment, your doctor will check your blood counts with blood tests.

Mouth Sores

Fortunately, mouth sores are a less common side effect of chemotherapy for lung cancer, but the treatment can cause painful sores and ulcers on the lips, in the mouth, on the gums, and inside the throat. The medical term for such mouth sores is *stomatitis*. In addition to discomfort, mouth sores may make eating and drinking difficult, which may lead to dehydration. In some instances, these sores become infected, and if they do occur, the sores disappear once the treatments have concluded.

If you do develop mouth sores, ask your doctor about medication to treat the sores. Here are additional suggestions for coping with mouth sores:

- If possible, have your teeth cleaned and any dental work completed before starting chemotherapy.
- Practice good oral hygiene—brush and floss regularly.
- Use a soft-bristle brush to avoid irritating gum tissue.
- Avoid mouthwashes that contain a lot of salt or alcohol.
- Stay hydrated by drinking plenty of water.

- Try sucking on ice chips; it may be soothing.
- Avoid spicy, sauce-based foods.
- Eat soft foods, such as baby food, cooled oatmeal, mashed vegetables, yogurt, ice cream, milk shakes, and smoothies.
- Try this homemade gargle: Mix one-half teaspoon of salt and one teaspoon of baking soda in one quart of water, and gargle every four hours.

If you do have mouth sores as a result of chemotherapy, they will heal after your treatment ends.

Diarrhea

Diarrhea is not one of the most common side effects for those undergoing chemotherapy for lung cancer; however, it can occur. It is caused by chemotherapy acting on the lining on the inside of the stomach and intestines. Abdominal cramping can also accompany diarrhea. Both may last several hours to several days. The concern about diarrhea is that, if not treated, it can lead to dehydration. If diarrhea becomes severe, you may need to have fluids replaced intravenously; hospitalization may be required.

Since diarrhea can cause the body to lose a large amount of water in a short period of time, you can also lose important minerals and electrolytes. If you're having diarrhea, take these measures:

- Drink at least six to eight glasses of water daily.
- Avoid high-fiber, greasy, and spicy foods.
- Eat small amounts of solid food frequently throughout the day.
- Avoid coffee, tea, alcohol, and sugary foods.

If diarrhea persists for more than twenty-four hours, contact your doctor. Do not take any over-the-counter medication for diarrhea without consulting your doctor.

Memory and Thinking Impairments

Some people have temporary changes in their memory and thinking process as a side effect of chemotherapy. Sometimes referred to as "brain fog," these impairments are usually mild, but can be frustrating. You might feel confused, have problems concentrating, or have trouble finding the word you want to use to express yourself. This side effect may linger from months to years. The severity of it depends on how much chemotherapy was given and the length of time it was given.

If you find yourself coping with memory and thinking impairments, here are steps you can take:

- Keep a notepad handy to make notes to yourself.
- Keep a calendar nearby for scheduling appointments and events.
- Get plenty of rest.
- Ask for support from family members and friends.

Some patients use exercise, music therapy, art, or reading to help them overcome memory and thinking impairments; however, it has not yet been scientifically proven that these activities are effective in overcoming such impairments.

Hand-Foot Syndrome

Chemotherapy may also cause a side effect called *hand-foot syndrome.* This syndrome occurs when small amounts of chemotherapy leak out of small blood vessels and cause damage to the surrounding tissues. Symptoms typically show up in the hands and feet and include redness, swelling, blisters, and flaking skin. If symptoms become severe, they can impair hand function and walking.

Your doctor will likely prescribe topical ointments for this condition. Here are other measures that may help:

- Limit the use of hot water on your hands and feet.
- Take cool baths.
- Pat skin dry after bathing; do not rub skin.
- Use ice packs for no more than fifteen minutes at a time; never apply ice directly to skin—wrap the ice in

a cloth.

- Apply skin care creams as recommended by your doctor.
- Avoid exposure to direct sunlight.
- Avoid activities such as brisk exercise that may cause clothing to rub against skin.

Although hand-foot syndrome typically affects hands and/ or feet, it can also occur on the elbows and knees.

Rash

Another potential side effect of some chemotherapy agents is an acnelike rash called *acneiform rash*. This rash may appear around the nose or elsewhere on the face, on the chest, or on the back. Your physician may prescribe antibiotic pills or topical gels to treat the rash. Over-the-counter medications to relieve itching may also be recommended.

Changes in the Skin and Nails

Changes can occur in the skin and nails during chemotherapy. Skin reactions may include drying, cracking, or peeling. Skin may also become *hyperpigmented*, or darkened. This may happen all over the body or just in spots. When a change in skin color occurs, it usually appears about two to three weeks after chemotherapy treatment begins. When treatment ends, the discoloration usually goes away as new skin cells grow. Sometimes, however, the darkening is permanent. It's important to wear sunblock to protect the skin when exposed to sunlight.

Nails may also become discolored. In addition, depressions may develop in both the fingernails and toenails. After treatment is over and the nails resume normal growth, these depressions and discoloration should disappear.

Allergic Reactions

Allergic reactions to chemotherapy agents are not common, but they can occur. Symptoms of an allergic reaction include shortness of breath, wheezing, hoarseness, swelling, hives, and itching. These symptoms may occur within seconds of beginning a treatment, or they may occur a few hours or days later. If a reaction occurs when you are not at your treatment center, contact your physician immediately. More severe allergic reactions may lower blood pressure or cause heart attack, shock, or loss of consciousness. Medications can be given to counteract allergic reactions.

If you have an allergic reaction to a chemotherapy agent, your oncologist will switch you to a different chemotherapy agent.

Infertility

If you are still in your childbearing years, chemotherapy for lung cancer may affect fertility. This side effect is rare, but it is possible for women to have damage to their ovaries and for men to have damage to the delicate lining of the testicles where sperm is produced. Among those whose fertility is affected, some women and men are eventually able to conceive; others are not. You'll want to speak with your oncologist if infertility is an issue for you.

Damage to the Liver and Kidneys

Chemotherapy drugs may cause damage to the liver and kidneys. The liver's primary function is to filter toxic substances from the body. If the liver is damaged, these toxins can build up and cause more liver damage. However, once chemotherapy is stopped, other drugs can be given to lessen the effects of liver damage.

The kidneys filter waste from the blood. It's not common, but chemotherapy can damage the blood vessels in the kidneys, causing them to malfunction. This malfunction is called *acute renal failure*. Fortunately, kidney damage is usually reversible. When chemotherapy is stopped, other measures can be taken to clear toxins from the blood, allowing the kidneys time to recover.

Those who have liver or kidney disease are generally not good candidates for chemotherapy, because the treatment can further damage these organs.

After Chemotherapy

After you complete your chemotherapy, your medical oncologist will want to see you for follow-up examinations. As part of the follow up, you'll have blood tests, X-rays, and scans.

Your oncologist will also want to monitor any side effects that are likely to linger such as fatigue, neuropathy, and thinking and memory impairments. Report these side effects, as well as any other problems, to your medical oncologist during your follow-up visits.

8 Clinical Trials

Should you participate in a lung cancer clinical trial? Perhaps you're not familiar enough with them to make an informed decision. To help you better understand clinical trials as a treatment option, this chapter will explain how they work.

A clinical trial is a research study conducted with patients in an attempt to find new and better treatments. In the field of cancer research, one of the goals of such a trial is to compare a new treatment to a standard treatment. Sometimes, it's recommended that treatment through a clinical trial be part of initial treatment. Other times, a clinical trial is recommended when initial treatment has failed to help.

It is important to remember that participants in clinical trials do not receive untested treatments. Many people mistakenly think that participating in a clinical trial makes them part of an unreliable experiment. However, treatments in these trials are offered only after extensive laboratory research has demonstrated that they are at least as good as, and potentially much better than, standard therapies.

The knowledge gained from clinical trials accounts for much of the progress that has been made in treating patients with cancer. Many of today's best standard treatments were first available to patients in clinical trials.

How Clinical Trials Work

After researchers identify a promising new treatment, the researchers, along with doctors, write a study plan, called a *protocol,* for a clinical trial of that treatment. The new treatment might involve a new anticancer drug, a new combination of treatment methods, or a new method for cancer prevention. The study plan is designed to safeguard the health of participants and answer research questions. It lists the types of people who may participate in the trial, along with information such as the schedule of tests, procedures, medications, dosages, and the length of the study.

Before a clinical trial can be offered to patients, an institutional review board (IRB) must approve the protocol for the organization, cancer center, hospital, clinic, or medical school where the trial will be conducted. The review board includes doctors, researchers, and members of the public.

The review board follows strict ethical guidelines for the conduct of medical research supported by both the federal government and the international community. The Food and Drug Administration (FDA) and the Office of Protection from Research Risks (OPRR) periodically review the conduct of the review board. The review board periodically monitors the results of the clinical trial to make sure that ethical practices are followed.

Types of Clinical Trials

There are several types of clinical trials, according to the National Institutes of Health. They include the following:

- *Treatment trials* test experimental treatments, new combinations of drugs, or new approaches to surgery or radiation therapy.
- *Prevention trials* seek better ways to prevent disease in people who have never had the disease or ways to prevent a disease from recurring. The approaches may include medicines, vaccines, vitamins, minerals, or lifestyle changes.
- *Diagnostic trials* are conducted to find better tests or procedures for diagnosing a disease or condition.
- *Screening trials* test the best way to detect certain diseases.
- *Quality-of-life trials* explore ways to improve comfort and the quality of life for individuals with chronic illnesses.

Participating in a Clinical Trial

Participation in a clinical trial is strictly voluntary. You may stop participating in a clinical trial at any time before, during, or after you have received the new treatment. Upon leaving the trial, if any medical problems result from the trial treatment, you will continue to receive appropriate medical care.

How do you enroll in a trial? Ask your doctor or oncologist to help you find a trial that is suitable. He or she will ask you to sign a consent form after reviewing all the details of the clinical trial with you, including the potential benefits and risks.

Clinical trials are offered in hospitals, cancer centers, doctors' offices, and clinics throughout the United States and internationally. However, some trials are available only at certain locations.

Phases of a Clinical Trial

Among the goals of clinical trials are determining whether a new drug or treatment is safe and determining optimal dosages. To this end, there are four phases of a clinical trial. After the experimental drug or treatment has tested well in one phase, more people are included in the next phase. The National Institutes of Health describes the four phases as follows.

- *Phase I:* Researchers test an experimental drug or treatment in a small group of people (20 to 80) for the first time, to evaluate its safety, determine a safe dosage range, and identify side effects.
- *Phase II:* The experimental study drug or treatment is given to a larger group of people (100 to 300) to determine whether it is effective and to further evaluate its safety.
- *Phase III:* The experimental drug or treatment is given to a large group of people (1,000 to 3,000) to confirm its effectiveness, monitor side effects, compare it to commonly used treatments, and collect information that will allow the experimental drug or treatment to be used safely.

- *Phase IV:* The new drug or treatment is studied after it has received FDA approval to be sold. Additional information about the risks and benefits of the drug or treatment is collected.

Advantages of Clinical Trials

- Participants receive a new therapy that is likely to produce better results than standard treatments.
- Participants are among the first to receive the new therapy.
- Responses to the new therapy, including side effects, are carefully monitored by doctors who specialize in cancer treatment.
- Participants contribute to the development of new treatments that may help others.

Disadvantages of Clinical Trials

- The new treatment may not prove more effective than standard treatments.
- Side effects of the new treatment may be unexpected or more severe than expected.
- Some costs of the treatment given during the clinical trial may not be covered by participants' insurance companies.
- Participants may have to travel a long distance to a specialized center to participate in the trial, as the new treatment may not be available everywhere.

Questions to Ask before Participating in a Clinical Trial

How does the new treatment that I might receive in the clinical trial differ from the standard treatments for my condition? This is an important question to ask your physician. You should have some idea of the rationale behind the new treatment—why doctors and researchers think it might be better.

Who may participate in the clinical trial? What are the eligibility criteria? Remember, however, that being turned down for a clinical trial does not mean that you cannot get better with the new treatment; it simply means that you aren't the type of patient for which the trial was designed.

What are the potential risks if I agree to participate? How will the treatment affect me physically or affect my day-to-day life? Answers to these questions are usually spelled out in the informed consent form that you must sign before participating. Be sure that you understand what the form says. If you don't understand it at first, don't hesitate to ask someone to explain it to you.

How long will the proposed treatment take? How many weeks or months? How many visits per week? Will I have to travel to another facility or another city for any part of the treatment? Once you have the answers to these questions, be realistic regarding your willingness to make the commitment required to participate in the trial.

Will the cost of any treatments or special tests required by the clinical trial be covered by my insurance? Your insurance plan may not cover all the costs because it may consider clinical trials to be experimental therapy. In many cases, the organization sponsoring the trial will cover the costs. Be sure to ask.

Finding Clinical Trials

As mentioned earlier, one of your doctors may recommend a clinical trial or help you find one. If you wish to research cancer clinical trials online, the National Cancer Institute provides a list at www.cancer.gov/clinicaltrials. The National Institutes of Health also lists clinical trials for cancer and other diseases on its Web site, www.clinicaltrials.gov.

9 Coping Emotionally

If you have been diagnosed with lung cancer, you already know how waves of emotions—fear, anger, anxiety—can surge through you. These emotions are tough enough to cope with. If you've been a smoker, you may also find yourself dealing with a stigma—the underlying belief that because you smoked, you are responsible for the disease. You may feel that friends and relatives blame you for getting lung cancer. Consequently, you may be experiencing feelings of isolation and abandonment.

It's a lot to deal with at a time when what you need most from those around you is love and support.

Smoker's Guilt

After a lung cancer diagnosis, smokers are often angry at themselves. In addition to blaming themselves for getting cancer, they may feel guilty for having caused emotional pain for their loved ones. Their guilt may also arise from concern over medical expenses and inconveniences to others. There is often a general feeling of having done wrong—a feeling of hopelessness and helplessness. Smokers experiencing such guilt should remember the following:

- Nicotine addiction is powerful. For many people, it's difficult to quit smoking. The fact that you didn't quit does not mean you are a weak person.
- You had no intentions of bringing disease upon yourself when you started smoking.
- Smoking was an easy habit to start. You may have

started smoking because of peer pressure. Perhaps you wanted to fit in, to belong to a circle of friends.
- There may be other reasons why you smoked. Perhaps it was a way of relaxing or of coping with anxiety. Maybe it increased your alertness.
- Cancer may strike anyone. No one asks for it.

In short, you didn't knowingly choose to cause your cancer. Now is the time to lighten your load of self-doubt, self-criticism, and guilt for whatever you feel you have done wrong. If you have a sense that you have done something wrong, forgive yourself, just as you might have forgiven others at times in your life.

And don't forget that support is available for dealing with these feelings. Don't fall into the isolation trap—it has a way of amplifying negative emotions.

Stress Management

Few things are more stressful than a diagnosis of cancer. Reducing stress has a powerful influence on the body. Increasing numbers of studies on the mind/body relationship demonstrate the connections between our thoughts, feelings, attitudes, and beliefs as they affect our behaviors, immune system, and overall physiology.

A strong immune system, of course, is necessary to resist infection, illness, and disease. Chronic psychological stress seems to be immunosuppressive, meaning it hampers the immune system's ability to function optimally.

It has been shown that stressful life events, particularly negative changes like divorce, bereavement, and other major losses, can increase the risk of developing diseases of any kind. Research continues on the relationship between stress and cancer. Studies with animals have shown that chronic stress impairs the ability of cells to repair structural damage, which is believed to influence the onset of cancer.

When we experience significant stress we become susceptible to the damaging effects of *cortisol*, a stress hormone that, in excessive amounts, may weaken the immune system.

Stress has varying effects on individuals according to their personality, coping skills, life circumstances, and the availability of social support. Developing effective stress management skills is particularly important for someone with cancer, who requires a strong immune system. Stress management skills may be learned and developed with practice.

Eliminate Stressors

Stress management begins by first assessing your stress level. Review the major negative stress factors in your life and eliminate as many as you can. In this way, you can free up more of your energy to deal effectively with what is most important now. Ask yourself what matters most in life. Put yourself at the top of your priority list. A certain amount of self-centeredness is required for optimal self-care. Practice saying "yes" to yourself and "no" to others when it is better to do so.

Identify things that drain your energy and eliminate as many as possible. Replace them with the things that fill you up, those people and activities that enliven you. Remember to pursue what is fun and what makes you laugh. These positive emotions will help balance the more serious aspects of life with an illness.

Get Adequate Nutrition, Sleep, and Exercise

Stress management includes making sure you have a nutritious diet that is low in sugar, caffeine, and processed foods. Good nutrition provides the nutrients that help to repair the body. The need for getting adequate sleep cannot be underestimated in helping you cope with stress. Adequate exercise may release toxic stress hormones stored in the body and stimulate *endorphins,* or "feel-good" hormones. Discuss any physical limitations of exercise with your doctor.

Practice Deep Breathing

Relaxation audiotapes, CD's, or digital downloads may be useful in stress management. Basic, deep abdominal breathing is effective at reducing anxiety. A simple, but effective, exercise is to close your eyes and take a deep breath, seeing yourself filled with vitality and peace and healing. As you exhale, imagine that you are also releasing any tension or negative feelings.

Touch

Touch is a remarkable stress reducer. Hold the hand of someone you love. Allow your loved ones to touch you in loving ways. Get as many hugs in a day as you can. It's okay to ask for a hug if you need one. Cuddling a pet works, too. Body massages can be very soothing, both physically and emotionally.

Express Emotions

Lung cancer patients often withdraw and suffer alone, which can intensify emotions and inhibit healing. Hiding deep feelings such as fear and sadness only makes us feel more stressed. Many of us have been trained to withhold our emotions; however, human feelings have a purpose. They serve as messengers, signaling a need to reevaluate or correct a situation. Feelings help us make the best choices. If we are reluctant to openly express emotion, our bodies may pay the price. During this time, don't look at your feelings as being right or wrong. They are simply feelings—part of being human.

Learning new ways to express feelings may be especially helpful for smokers. For some, smoking is a temporary fix for difficult or uncomfortable feelings such as anger, worry, loneliness, or fear. The smoking habit can keep a person from learning other, more appropriate ways to experience and resolve situations that evoke strong emotional responses.

Social Support

Social support during a life crisis can be powerful. Support groups can help you learn about both your condition and ways to cope with it. Perhaps most importantly, support groups can relieve feelings of loneliness and isolation. You can learn that you are not alone in your journey—that many others are taking the same journey.

Support groups allow people to communicate with other people who are living with cancer, providing a safe setting to discuss a variety of issues related to having cancer. The groups usually focus on daily living, relationships, and communication problems; they provide a place to discuss subjects or feelings you may not wish to share with loved ones or friends.

Numerous studies have shown that people with social support have lower mortality rates from a variety of diseases compared to those without support. Cancer patients with stronger social support may actually live longer than patients with weaker social support. Solid support systems are associated with both better adjustment and longer survival.

How strong is your social support system? How connected do you feel to other people? You may have chosen a life of isolation in order to feel safe. If so, you may find yourself painfully lonely now, during a life crisis. We all need others. We are interdependent. It is okay to reach out, even though it may feel awkward at first.

You may want to think about the important people in your life. Who accepts you for who you are? Who do you trust completely? Who shows an interest in your well-being? Who has coped with similar problems? Who could help you with daily activities? Who could be there for you if you opened up more and nurtured that relationship? Serving the needs of others and reciprocating good deeds are gifts for the givers, too.

You can stay in touch with family and friends through several online sites. These Web sites, listed in the Resources section at the back of this book, allow you to create private pages where you can post updates about your hospital stays and treatments without making multiple phone calls or sending e-mails.

Counseling

Counseling takes many forms. It includes individual psychotherapy, family therapy, group therapy, and support groups. Counseling may prove most beneficial for those who suspect they have powerful buried feelings that are affecting their ability to heal both physically and emotionally. It is possible to overcome feelings of self-blame, anger, anxiety, and depression and gain a renewed sense of well-being. People who have a positive sense of self-worth tend to take better care of themselves.

Individual counseling may help you evaluate the changes you need to make to improve the quality of your life. It may assist you, too, in expressing your feelings and needs with others, improving relationship dynamics, and becoming more assertive as needed with medical providers.

Family counseling may be helpful, too. There can be so much strain put on all family members when a major illness strikes. Effective family counseling can help us become stronger emotionally as individuals; it can also help us develop stronger relationships. Opening the channels for honest discussion and clarifying needs and feelings has united many families in the quest for healing. Facing feelings and problems courageously and honestly can be challenging; however, many families who have sought counseling report even more fulfilling lives than before they had to cope with cancer.

Fear of cancer recurrence is normal, but you need not carry extreme and unrealistic fears. Asking the questions you need answered to ease your worry is warranted. When it comes to taking good care of yourself, there are no "silly" questions. It is wiser to expend energy caring for yourself rather than worrying. Talking about your feelings with a family member or friend, your physician, or a support group can help you deal with troubling concerns and emotions. Let others know you need help.

Finding Support Services

Your health care team will likely have suggestions for you on where to find services for you and your family. You can also contact the National Cancer Institute. Information specialists will help you locate programs, services, and publications. You can speak with a specialist by calling 1-800-4-CANCER. Or you can interact with a specialist online by going online to www.cancer.gov. After you're on the site, do a search for "Live Help."

10 Smoking: It's Not Too Late to Quit

If you are a smoker who has been diagnosed with lung cancer, you have probably smoked for many years, and smoking has probably been an important part of your life. It may have helped you relieve stress or anxiety. As you know, nicotine is the addictive compound in tobacco smoke. It is absorbed into the bloodstream and reaches the brain in seconds. There, it stimulates the release of chemicals that affect the brain's pleasure centers.

Whatever your reason for smoking, you also know how difficult it is to quit. Smoking becomes an addiction. And, if you have tried to give up smoking before, you know how strong and powerful this addiction is. In fact, many people who develop lung cancer continue to smoke after their diagnosis.

However, there is still good reason to quit.

Why Quit Now?

We've all heard that smoking is hazardous to our health. Tobacco smoke contains carbon monoxide, the same gas found in automobile exhaust. The carbon monoxide attaches to the body's red blood cells in place of oxygen; this deprives the heart and the rest of the body of oxygen. Other compounds in tobacco smoke cause blood platelets to become stickier, increasing the likelihood of blood clots. Even though you may feel it's too late to quit, you can still benefit from giving up smoking. Anything that makes breathing harder—such as smoking—doesn't help.

71

Improve Your Response
to Cancer Treatment

Continuing to smoke increases the likelihood of developing complications from lung cancer treatments—surgery, radiation therapy, and chemotherapy. For example, after surgery, smokers more often suffer lung problems such as pneumonia. They usually have more mucus to cough up after surgery and may have a more difficult time doing so. They may have to spend more time on a ventilator or in the hospital.

How well a person does with radiation therapy or chemotherapy is related to his or her overall health. Smoking may intensify therapy-related fatigue and contribute to a decrease in appetite; it may also worsen chemotherapy-related nausea. It helps to do all you can to improve your overall health condition.

Cancer treatments that are designed to eliminate cancer cells inevitably damage some normal lung tissues as well as other tissues. This is often true with surgery, when some surrounding lung tissue must be removed in order to extract all of the cancer. This is also true of radiation therapy. New treatment plans minimize the amount of normal lung tissue affected by the radiation beams, but some normal tissue is still damaged. Therefore, it makes sense to quit smoking and conserve as much functioning lung as you can.

View smoking cessation as part of your cancer treatment. Quitting smoking will increase your chances of responding well to treatment.

Stop Smoking to Prevent
Other Medical Problems

As mentioned, smoking contributes to the blood platelets becoming sticky, potentially causing the formation of blood clots. If a clot forms in a blood vessel that carries oxygen to the heart muscle, a heart attack may occur. If a clot forms in a blood vessel in the brain, a stroke may occur. Smoking can also cause *emphysema*, a progressive loss of functional lung tissue. Progressive emphysema leads to breathlessness.

Quitting smoking dramatically slows the further loss of lung function.

Quitting smoking may also help prevent the development of a second lung cancer in another part of the affected lung or in your other lung. The precancerous changes that eventually turned into a cancerous tumor in one area may also be present in other parts of your lungs. Continued exposure to smoke may produce another cancer. Research has shown that patients with a successfully treated early-stage lung cancer (stage I, II, and some stage III) have a 2 to 3 percent chance per year of developing another lung cancer. If you continue to smoke, the likelihood of developing a second lung cancer is even greater.

Develop a Plan to Quit

There is not just one "correct" way to quit smoking. Find a method that works best for you. Some people simply make the decision to quit and never touch tobacco again. However, for most people, it is much more difficult to quit and requires some planning. Smoking cessation experts recommend picking a "quit date." It's a matter of choice whether you decide to gradually smoke fewer cigarettes until your quit date or whether you plan to smoke until that day and then go "cold turkey."

Many smokers first resolve to quit while they are in the hospital following surgery or other treatment for lung cancer. This is an excellent time to quit. You are in a supportive environment; doctors (and nurses) are available to answer your questions and to prescribe smoking cessation drugs.

It is probably easier to not smoke while in the hospital than it will be at home. The hospital is a different environment without all the smoking triggers that you are accustomed to. Take some time while in the hospital to think about smoking triggers—specific events that make you crave a cigarette.

Identify Triggers

What are your triggers to light a cigarette? Do you like to smoke while talking on the telephone? After a meal? Or when having that first cup of coffee in the morning? Do smoke breaks give you time to talk to friends at work? Once you have identified some of these smoking triggers, you can think about how to respond when they come up in the course of daily life. Decide how you will handle them effectively.

Remember, the desire to light a cigarette usually lasts only three to five minutes. Experts recommend coming up with a list of things to do other than smoking when your craving hits. Take a walk if you can, drink water, do some breathing exercises, or practice stress management. Suck on hard candy or "puff" on a straw; keep your hands busy. And don't be surprised if you crave cigarettes long after you quit smoking. Smoking is a complex behavior that involves more than simply the body craving nicotine.

Participate in a Smoking Cessation Program

Participating in a smoking cessation program can be of enormous benefit. If you have been diagnosed with lung cancer, you already have a lot to deal with emotionally, and you may appreciate help from a smoking cessation program. The best results are usually obtained by participating in a comprehensive program, one that includes all the components currently recommended by the U.S. Agency for Health Care Policy and Research (AHCPR). This agency views tobacco dependence as a chronic disease and recommends strategies to help people quit smoking. These strategies include education, emotional support, smoking cessation medications, and relapse prevention training.

Choose a program that emphasizes how to change your behavior, and consider seeing a counselor to support your efforts. Many people benefit from participating in both individual counseling and support groups. Also, numerous "quit lines" are also available. These are help lines you can call to speak to counselors about quitting. You can find these quit lines by doing an online search.

Drug therapy is an important component of a smoking cessation program. Nicotine replacement drugs and other medications have proved effective in helping smokers quit.

Drug Therapy

Drug therapy plays an important role in smoking cessation. There are two types of drugs that help people quit smoking: nicotine replacements and prescription medications that do not contain nicotine. Both are designed to ease symptoms of withdrawal, such as irritability, frustration, anger, anxiety, difficulty concentrating, restlessness, and depression.

Nicotine Gum

Nicotine polacrilex, better known as *nicotine gum,* is a nicotine replacement that is available over the counter. Basic instructions call for chewing the gum slowly until you feel a mild tingling, which is the nicotine being released. Then "park" the gum between your cheek and gums for several minutes before chewing it again. This technique provides for gradual absorption of the nicotine and should continue for thirty minutes per piece of gum. Most people find that ten to fifteen pieces of gum per day are needed initially in order to successfully quit smoking. Nicotine lozenges that dissolve in your mouth are also available.

Nicotine Patches

Nicotine patches, which must be obtained by a prescription from your physician, resemble adhesive bandages and are applied to the skin. The sticky side of the patch contains a layer of nicotine that passes through the skin into your blood. The directions recommend choosing a different, hairless site somewhere above the waist each time a patch is replaced.

You should not exceed the recommended dosage unless supervised by your physician. However, your doctor may prescribe a higher dosage (wearing more than one patch at a time) if you are a heavy smoker. Side effects include mild skin irritation at the site of the patch.

Many smokers worry about receiving too much nicotine from a patch, especially if they smoke while wearing one. However, smokers get much higher levels of nicotine in their

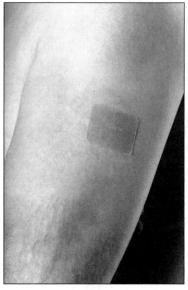

A popular smoking cessation aid, the nicotine patch provides a steady controlled dose of nicotine throughout the day, reducing nicotine withdrawal.

blood from smoking compared to what they receive from a nicotine patch. So, don't let this concern keep you from using a nicotine patch that might help you quit smoking.

Nicotine Nasal Spray

Nicotine nasal spray is a nicotine replacement. Sold under the brand name *Nicotrol,* this spray works by delivering nicotine to your body through the nostrils. It is sprayed against the lower nasal lining; it should not be sprayed or sniffed into the upper nasal passages. Most people use about fifteen doses per day and gradually decrease the number of doses over time. Most individuals can use the spray successfully for up to twelve weeks.

Side effects may include runny nose, throat irritation, watering eyes, sneezing, coughing, and a hot, peppery feeling in the nose or the back of the throat.

Nicotine Inhaler

A *nicotine inhaler* resembles a cigarette and contains a small capsule filled with nicotine-treated cotton. Puffing on the device delivers vaporized nicotine to the linings of the mouth and upper throat where it is absorbed. It may be the best choice for anyone who needs the ritual or "feel" of smoking. Unlike a nicotine patch, which delivers a constant level of nicotine, a nicotine inhaler produces a more rapid increase in nicotine levels in the blood, followed by a decrease in nicotine levels—more like an actual cigarette.

Possible side effects include mild irritation of the mouth or throat, cough, upset stomach, nausea, diarrhea, and hiccups.

Zyban

The prescription drug *Zyban* is the brand name for the drug *bupropion*. It was the first medication approved by the Food and Drug Administration (FDA) for smoking cessation. It comes in pill form and does not contain nicotine. The drug helps reduce withdrawal symptoms and stimulates the release of the same brain chemicals released in response to nicotine. These chemicals improve alertness, concentration, and memory. Also, by stimulating pleasure centers in the brain, the drug also simulates some of the other effects of nicotine. Patients are usually instructed to continue smoking for two weeks after starting Zyban to allow a level of the drug to build up in the body before the planned quit date.

> **When You Decide to Quit**
>
> - Set a definite "quit date."
> - Dispose of all tobacco, lighters, and ashtrays.
> - Let someone else know about your plan—someone who can help you stay accountable to yourself.
> - Ask your doctor about medications that can help treat nicotine withdrawal.
> - Be prepared to handle cravings and to feel discomfort for the first week or two.
> - Expect to be less productive; plan a lighter workload.
> - Avoid situations that trigger smoking.
> - Have low-calorie snacks available.
> - Quit for one day at a time.
> - Reward yourself for your success.
> - If you slip, don't get discouraged. Start back on your plan.

Potential side effects of Zyban include anxiety, changes in appetite, constipation, diarrhea, dizziness, drowsiness, dry mouth, headache, increased sweating, nausea, nervousness, stomach pain, stuffy nose, trouble sleeping, vomiting, and weight changes.

Chantix

Chantix is the brand name for the non-nicotine drug *varenicline*. It works by blocking the pleasant effects of nicotine on the brain. The drug comes in pill form and is usually taken once or twice a day to start. It's recommended that you begin taking Chantix a week before you stop smoking completely. This gives the drug a chance to build up in your body. You may smoke during the first week of treatment, but you should stop smoking completely on the eighth day of treatment.

The most common side effects of Chantix are nausea, insomnia, constipation, gas, and vomiting. According to the patient information that comes with a prescription, anyone taking the drug should be observed for any psychological problems that may develop; there have been reports of depression and suicidal thoughts among those taking Chantix.

You Can Succeed!

It takes persistence and dedication to give up smoking. Smoking cessation experts say that most people make more than one serious attempt before actually quitting for good. It is important not to be discouraged by an occasional slip. When you do have a slip, try to understand what caused you to want to smoke. Plan to handle that situation differently next time. Then, set another quit date and try again.

Once you have quit, reward yourself. Remember, too, that you'll need to stay vigilant—remaining a nonsmoker requires effort. It may be a while before you stop *thinking* about having a cigarette.

11 A Closing Note

Just as being diagnosed with lung cancer was an event filled with emotion finishing cancer treatment can also be emotional. You may feel relief at having completed treatment, but you may also be worried about what lies ahead. In the back of your mind, you may be wondering, What if the cancer recurs? Once you stop seeing your health care team on a frequent basis, you might feel vulnerable. Each ache or pain you have may cause you to question whether you're having a recurrence of the cancer. It's normal to feel this way.

Meanwhile, the doctors who have been part of your health care team will want to monitor you closely after you complete treatment. Typically, follow-up appointments will be scheduled at least every six months for the first two years after your treatment ends. Then, follow-up examinations will be performed once a year for three years. If you have had no recurrence after five years, you are considered cured of the cancer.

If you should have a recurrence, your treatment plan will again depend on factors such as the location of the cancer, the nature of the tumor, and your overall health. As before, treatments may include surgery, radiation therapy, and chemotherapy. If you receive additional treatments, you'll have a better idea of what to expect as you work with healthcare team.

Appendix

TNM Classification System

Doctors use an internationally recognized system for classifying the extent to which a cancer has spread. Known as the "TNM" classification system, it has been accepted by the International Union Against Cancer (UICC) and the American Joint Committee on Cancer (AJCC).

In the initials, TNM, the "**T**" stands for tumor—its size and the extent of any spreading. The "**N**" is for lymph nodes and refers to any spread of the cancer to lymph nodes. The "**M**" is for metastasis or spread to other organs. Descriptions of the system are listed below. If you wish to learn more about this staging system, talk to your oncologist.

Primary Tumor (T)	
Tx	Primary tumor cannot be assessed , or tumor proven by the presence of malignant cells in sputum or bronchial washings but not visualized by imaging orbronchoscopy.
T0	No evidence of primary tumor.
Tis	Carcinoma in situ:
T1	Tumor 3 cm or less in greatest dimension, surrounded by lung or visceral pleura, without bronchoscopic evidence of invasion more proximal than the lobar bronchus (for example, not in the main bronchus).
T1a	Tumor 2 cm or less in greatest dimension.
T1b	Tumor more than 2 cm but 3 cm or less in greatest dimension.

T2	Tumor more than 3 cm but 7 cm or less or tumor with any of the following features (T2 tumors with these features are classified T2a if 5 cm or less): involves main bronchus, 2 cm or more distal to the carina; invades visceral pleura (PL1 or PL2); associated with atelectasis or obstructive pneumonitis that extends to the hilar region but does not involve the entire lung.
T2a	Tumor more than 3 cm but 5 cm or less in greatest dimension.
T2b	Tumor more than 5 cm but 7 cm or less in greatest dimension.
T3	Tumor more than 7 cm or one that directly invades of any of the following: Parietal pleural (PL3), chest wall (including superior sulcus tumors), diaphragm, phrenic nerve, mediastinal pleura, parietal pericardium; or tumor in the main bronchus less than 2 cm distal to the carina but without involvement of the carina; or associated atelectasis or obstructive pneumonitis of the entire lung or separate tumor nodule(s) in the same lobe.
T4	Tumor of any size that invades of the follow: medastinum, heart, great vessels, trachea, recurrent laryngeal nerve, esophagus, vertebral body, carina, separate tumor nodules(s) in a different ipsilateral lobe.
Regional Lymph Notes (N)	
NX	Region lymph nodes cannot be assessed.
N0	No regional lymph node metastases.
N1	Metastasis in ipsilaterail peribronchial and/or ipsilateral hilar lymph nodes and intrapulmonary nodes, including involvement by direct extension.
N2	Metastasis in ipsilateral mediastinal and/or subcarinal lymph node(s).
N3	Metastasis in contralateral mediastinal, contralateral hilar, ipsilateral or contralateral scalene, or supraclavicular lymph nodes.

Distant Metastasis (M)	
M0	No distant metastasis.
M1	Distant metastasis.
M1a	M1a Separate tumor nodules(s) in a contralateral lobe, tumor with pleural nodes or malignant pleural (or pericardial) effusion.
M1b	Distant metastasis (in extrathoracic organs).

Anatomic Stage/Prognostic Groups			
Occult Carcinoma	**TX**	**N0**	**M0**
Stage 0	Tis	N0	M0
Stage I A	T1a	N0	M0
	T1b	N0	M0
Stage I B	T2a	N0	M0
Stage II A	T2b	N0	M0
	T1a	N1	M0
	T1b	N1	M0
	T2a	N1	M0
Stage II B	T2b	N1	M0
	T3	N0	M0
Stage III A	T1a	N2	M0
	T1b	N2	M0
	T2a	N2	M0
	T2b	N2	M0

	T3	N1	M0
	T3	N2	M0
	T4	N0	M0
	T4	N1	M0
Stage III B			
	T1a	N3	M0
	T1b	N3	M0
	T2a	N3	M0
	T2b	N3	M0
	T3	N3	M0
	T4	N2	M0
	T4	N3	M0
Stage IV			
	Any T	Any N	M1a
	Any T	Any N	M1b

Resources

American Cancer Society
15999 Clifton Road NE
Atlanta, GA 30329-4251
(800) 227-2345
www.cancer.org

American Lung Association
1301 Pennsylvania Avenue NW, Suite 800,
Washington, DC 20004
(800) LUNG USA
www.lungusa.org

CancerCare
275 Seventh Avenue, 22nd Floor
New York, NY 10001
(800) 813 HOPE (4673)
www.cancercare.org
www.lungcancer.org

Cancer.Net
c/o American Society of Clinical Oncology
2318 Mill Road, Suite 800
Alexandria, VA 22314
(888) 651-3038
www.cancer.net

Lung Cancer Alliance
888 16th Street, NW, Suite 150
Washington, DC 20006
(800) 298-2436
www.lungcanceralliance.org

Lung Cancer Caring Ambassadors Program
www.lungcancercap.org

Lung Cancer Online Foundation
www.lungcanceronline.org

LUNGevity Foundation
435 North LaSalle Street, Suite 310
Chicago, IL 60654
(312) 464-0716
www.lungevity.org

MedlinePlus: Lung Cancer
National Institutes of Health
8600 Rockville Pike
Bethesda, MD 20894
www.medlineplus.gov/lungcancer

National Cancer Institute
Office of Communications and Education
Public Inquiries Office
6116 Executive Boulevard, Suite 300
Bethesda, MD 20892-8322
(800) 4-CANCER
www.cancer.gov

National Lung Cancer Partnership
222 North Midvale Boulevard, Suite 6
Madison, WI 53705
(608) 233-7905
www.nationallungcancerpartnership.org

Staying Connected to Family and Friends

The following are Web sites where you can post private health updates.

CareFlash
www.careflash.com

CarePages
www.carepages.com

CaringBridge
www.caringbridge.org

Family Patient
www.familypatient.com

Lotsa Helping Hands
www.lotsahelpinghands.com

MyLifeLine.org
www.mylfeline.org

The Status
www.thestatus.com

Glossary

A

Anesthesiologist: A physician who specializes in the administration of anesthesia.

Anhidrosis: An abnormal absence of sweat production on a certain area of the skin.

Anorexia: Loss of appetite for food.

Arterial blood gas: A blood test that provides information about lung function.

Asbestos: A mineral fiber once used in insulation that when inhaled increases the risk that a person developing lung cancer.

B

Biopsy: Surgical removal of a portion or all of a mass or organ.

Blood count: A test that counts the number of different cells that are contained in the blood.

Bone marrow: Tissue contained within the center of bones that makes the blood cells.

Bone scan: A test that can identify if cancer has spread to bone.

Brachytherapy: Radiation treatment that uses radioactive pellets inserted into a flexible tube placed inside the breathing passage to directly treat a lung cancer.

Bronchial basal epithelial cells: Cells that line the breathing passages, a common site where lung cancers develop.

Bronchial tree: The multiple airways and their branches contained within the lungs.

Bronchoalveolar carcinoma: One specific type of non-small cell lung cancer that can be diffuse, multicentric, or localized. If localized, surgical removal may be associated with a high cure rate.

Bronchoscope: Long, thin, flexible or rigid tube used to look into the breathing passages of the lung.

Bronchus: The main or large breathing passage in each lung.

C

Carbon dioxide: A by-product of normal body function, this waste gas is exhaled from the lungs.

Carcinogen: Any cancer-producing substance.

Carcinoma in situ: Cancer that is still confined to the area where it first developed.

CAT scan: Computerized axial tomography, or CT scan, an X-ray test that produces cross-sectional images of the body that are more detailed than standard X-rays.

Cervical mediastinoscopy: A procedure during which a thin tube is inserted through an incision above the breastbone in order to examine tissue in the area between the lungs.

Chemotherapy: The treatment of a disease, such as cancer, with chemical agents.

Chest tube: A flexible tube inserted between the ribs and into the space surrounding the lungs in order to drain air or fluid.

Chiropractic: A field of healing based on spinal manipulation and alignment.

Chronic obstructive pulmonary disease: A name for a number of long-term breathing problems with various causes such as aging and smoking.

Clavicle: The collarbone.

Community Clinical Oncology Program (CCOP): A program funded by the National Cancer Institute designed to make clinical trials available to patients in community hospitals.

Computerized tomography: See CAT scan.

Curative treatment: A treatment intended to eradicate disease.

D

Diagnostic radiologist: A medical specialist trained to read X-rays.

Diaphragm: A muscle located between the chest and the abdomen that helps with breathing.

Diarrhea: Liquid or watery stool.

Diffusion capacity: A test that helps to determine the amount of functioning lung tissue.

Dysphagia: Difficulty swallowing either solids or liquids.

Dysplasia: An increase in both the number of cells in a tissue and in the size of those cells; a precancerous change.

Dyspnea: Shortness of breath.

E

Emphysema: A condition affecting the lungs characterized by loss of functioning lung tissue and progressive shortness of breath.

Endorphins: Compounds made by the body that affect the perception of pain.

Esophagus: The muscular swallowing tube that connects the mouth and the stomach.

Excisional biopsy: Surgical removal of an entire mass in order to determine what it is.

Exercise treadmill test: A test that measures the heart and lung function of a person while they are walking on a treadmill.

Exploratory thoracotomy: Chest surgery that is performed when no clear preoperative diagnosis was possible.

Extensive : A term used to describe small cell lung cancer when it has spread beyond the chest.

External beam radiation therapy: Radiation therapy that is given by directing a beam of radiation at the cancer from a source located outside of the body.

F

Femur: The thigh bone.

Food and Drug Administration (FDA): The federal government agency that is responsible for approving new medical treatments.

G

General anesthetic: A state of unconsciousness produced by anesthetic agents.

Glucose: A sugar that is the chief source of energy for living organisms.

H

Hemoptysis: Coughing up any amount of blood.

Hemorrhoids: Veins near the anus that can become swollen and painful and sometimes bleed.

Horner syndrome: Symptoms (a small pupil, a droopy eyelid, and absence of sweating all on one side of the face) signifying dysfunction of the sympathetic nerve on that side of the body.

Hospice: A facility that provides supportive care to terminally ill patients and their families.

Hyperplasia: An abnormal increase in the number of cells in an otherwise normal tissue.

I

Immunosuppressant: An agent that diminishes or prevents the immune response.

Infection: Inflammation in body tissue caused by microorganisms.

Inflammation: A localized response to tissue injury characterized by swelling, redness, heat, tenderness, and loss of function.

Infusion: The therapeutic introduction of fluid or medicine into a vein.

Institutional review board: A group authorized to insure that research that involves humans is conducted according to ethical standards.

Interventional radiologist: A specialist trained to perform procedures, such as biopsies, using imaging equipment such as X-rays.

Intravenous: Administration of medication or fluid to a patient by introducing it through a vein.

L

Large cell carcinoma: A specific type of non-small cell lung cancer which may grow and spread more aggressively.

Laryngeal nerves: Nerves that activate the vocal cords.

Larynx: The voice box in the neck.

Lid lag: A droopy eyelid, one that moves more slowly when blinking.

Limited: A term that describes small cell lung cancer when it has not spread beyond the chest.

Liver: An organ located in the right upper part of the abdomen that has a number of important bodily functions. One of the organs that lung cancer can spread to.

Lobectomy: The surgical removal of one of the lobes of a lung.

Lobes: One of the main divisions of a lung.

Local anesthetic: A drug used to block sensation in a specific area of the body.

Low-dose spiral CT scan: A CT scan that uses fewer X-rays; used for early lung cancer detection.

Lymph nodes: Collections of lymph tissue located throughout the body, they are a source of lymphocytes that fight infection and cancer.

M

Magnetic resonance imaging (MRI): A machine that produces images of the body using magnetic fields.

Malignant tumor: A tumor that can invade tissue, grow uncontrollably, and spread to other tissues; a cancer.

Mediastinal lymph nodes: Lymph nodes located in the chest between the lungs, common site of lung cancer spread.

Mediastinoscope: Thin tube inserted into the mediastinum that doctors look through in order to view this area, biopsy lymph nodes, etc.

Mediastinum: That area between the lungs that contains the heart, the windpipe, the esophagus, lymph nodes, nerves, and blood vessels.

Medical oncologist: A specialist trained to use medicine to treat cancers.

Metastasis: An area of cancer that has spread from another part of the body.

Minimally invasive surgery: Surgery through small incisions, sometimes using television cameras to provide adequate vision for the surgeons.

Miosis: A smaller than normal (constricted) pupil.

Multimodality therapy: A treatment program that combines at least two of the three main methods for treating cancer: surgery, radiation therapy, or chemotherapy.

Mutation: A change in genetic material.

N

National Cancer Institute: U.S. government agency charged with promoting research and new treatment of cancer.

Needle biopsy: A procedure in which a needle is advanced through the chest into a tumor mass within or near the lung in order to obtain a small piece of the tumor.

Neoadjuvant therapy: Refers to treatments such as chemotherapy or combined chemotherapy and radiation therapy when they are given before surgical treatment.

Nerves: A fiber containing nerve cells that conveys impulses from the central nervous system to other parts of the body.

Neurologic: Referring to the nervous system.

Nicotine replacement therapy (NRT): Any of several methods of administering nicotine in order to minimize symptoms of withdrawal arising from smoking cessation.

Non-small cell lung cancer: The most common type of lung cancer, it accounts for 75-80% of all lung cancers.

O

Oncologist: A physician who specializes in the treatment of cancer patients.

P

Palliative treatment: Treatment administered with the goal of making the patient feel better or to improve function as opposed to destroying a cancer.

Pancoast syndrome: A collection of symptoms including pain in the arm and in the armpit, wasting of the arm muscles, and Horner syndrome caused by a lung cancer growing at the top of the lung.

Parietal pleura: The layer of tissue that lines the inside of the chest cavity.

Pathologist: A medical specialist trained to detect the structural changes in tissues and cells caused by disease.

Patient-controlled anesthesia (PCA): A device that allows the patient to self-administer safe amounts of pain medication.

Performance status: A way of describing the overall function of a person, a key indicator of response to chemotherapy.

Perfusion scan: A test that estimates the blood flow to each lung.

Pericardium: The sac that surrounds the heart.

Peripheral neuropathy: Functional disturbances of the peripheral nerves sometimes caused by chemotherapy, accounting for symptoms such as numbness and tingling sensations in the hands and toes.

Peripheral vascular disease: Hardening of the arteries occurring in blood vessels other than the heart.

Phrenic nerve: The nerve responsible for moving the diaphragm muscle during breathing, there is one nerve on each side of the chest.

Platelets: Cells in the blood that are important for blood clotting.

Pleura: The layer of cells covering the lungs and the inside of the chest cavity, the pleura surrounds the pleural space.

Pleural effusion: Fluid that has accumulated in the pleural space surrounding the lungs.

Pleuritic chest pain: Sharp, stabbing chest pain that occurs with breathing.

Pneumonectomy: The surgical removal of an entire lung.

Pneumonia: An infection within the lung.

Pneumothorax: Air that has accumulated in the pleural space.

Port: A device usually implanted under the skin that is used for the infusion of drugs or fluid into the bloodstream or for drawing blood for blood tests.

Positron emission tomography (PET): A test that produces an image based on the uptake of glucose by a cancer, used to determine if a tumor is a cancer and if a cancer has spread.

Prognosis: The likely outcome of a disease, often given in terms of the expected chance of surviving for a certain number of years.

Progressive muscle relaxation: A relaxation technique.

Prophylactic cranial irradiation: Radiation therapy to the brain in patients with small cell lung cancer to prevent brain metastases from developing.

Pulmonary artery: The blood vessel that brings blood that is depleted of oxygen to the lungs.

Pulmonary function tests: A general term for a number of breathing tests and blood tests that together measure lung function.

Pulmonary medicine specialist: A medical doctor trained in the diagnosis and treatment (with medicines) of lung and breathing disorders.

Pulmonary vein: The blood vessel that brings oxygenated blood from the lungs to the heart so that it can be pumped to the rest of the body.

Q

Quit date: The date chosen to stop smoking entirely.

R

Radiation oncologist: A medical doctor specializing in the treatment of cancer with radiation.

Radiation pneumonitis: Inflammation in the lung that sometimes results from the radiation therapy beam.

Radiation recall: The reoccurrence of a side effect of radiation treatments (such as skin irritation) long after the radiation therapy has been completed.

Radiation therapist: A specially trained technician who administers radiation treatments.

Radioactive seeds: Small pellets of radioactive material that can be placed down a catheter positioned in the breathing passage during brachytherapy.

Radon: A naturally occurring gas originating from the ground that when inhaled is associated with increased rates of lung cancer development.

Red blood cells: The cells in the blood that carry oxygen.

Resectable: The finding that a cancer does not grow into any vital structure and can therefore be removed by a surgical procedure.

Respiratory therapists: Specially trained technicians who monitor and maintain the respiratory status of patients.

S

Screening: The detection of a disease process before it causes any symptoms.

Segmentectomy: The smallest anatomically complete resection of the lung that can be performed.

Seizures: Convulsions or muscle spasms sometimes caused by spread of cancer to the brain.

Shortness of breath: The sensation of not being able to catch one's breath.

Side effects: A consequence of a treatment other than the one for which it was used.

Small cell lung cancer: One of the two main types of lung cancer, often widespread by the time it is diagnosed.

Sputum: Material brought up from the breathing passages.

Sputum cytology: Analysis of cells present in sputum to determine if there are signs of cancer.

Squamous cell carcinoma: One of the specific types of non-small cell lung cancer.

Stage: The anatomic extent of a cancer, how far it has spread.

Staging: The methods and procedures in determining the stage of a cancer.

Stroke: Sudden loss of brain function from bleeding, blood clot, or other injury.

Subclavian vein: Large vein behind the clavicle, sometimes used for infusion of fluid or medicine.

Submucosal gland cells: Cells that line the breathing passages where adenocarcinoma arises.

Superior vena cava: The large vein that drains blood from the head, neck, and arms back to the heart; may be blocked by a lung cancer in the upper right lung.

Superior vena cava syndrome: Swelling in the head, neck, and arms caused by obstruction of the superior vena cava by a lung cancer.

Surgeon: A medical doctor trained to perform surgery.

Survival: The act of continuing to live after a certain event, such as a diagnosis of lung cancer.

Symptom: A change in condition as perceived by a patient; subjective evidence of disease.

T

Thoracic surgeon: A surgeon who has undergone at least two additional years of training in order to specialize in heart and lung surgery.

Thoracotomy: General term for an operation on the chest using an incision made between the ribs.

Three-dimensional conformal radiation therapy: A special method of treating someone with external beam radiation therapy that minimizes exposure of normal tissue to radiation.

TNM: An abbreviation for tumor, lymph nodes, and metastases, a method of describing important features about a cancer.

Trachea: The windpipe.

Transfusion: The procedure of giving blood or blood products to a person.

Transthoracic needle aspiration biopsy: The technique of sticking a needle through the chest and into the lung or mediastinum for the purpose of taking a biopsy of a tumor or other mass.

Tumor: An abnormal mass or growth inside the body.

V

Video-assisted thoracoscopy (VATS): Minimally invasive surgery on the chest using a special television camera and special instruments.

Visceral pleura: The lining on the surface of the lung.

W

Wedge resection: a surgical procedure to remove a small piece of the lung.

Wheezing: Noisy breathing as a result of a partially obstructed breathing passage.

White blood cells: Cells in the blood that fight infection.

Wound infection: Infection of a surgical incision.

Index

About the Author

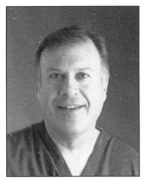

Walter J. Scott, M.D., F.A.C.S., is chief of the Division of Thoracic and Esophageal Surgery at Philadelphia's Fox Chase Cancer Center, one of the first National Cancer Institute–designated Comprehensive Cancer Centers. Board certified in thoracic surgery, Dr. Scott specializes in the treatment of cancers involving the chest, with a special emphasis on the treatment of lung cancer. He has been recognized as a Top Doctor in Philadelphia and as one of America's Top Doctors for Cancer Treatment (Thoracic Surgery) by Castle Connolly, Sixth Edition.

Dr. Scott's research interests include the use of positron emission tomography (PET) for the diagnosis and evaluation of patients with lung cancer and the development of minimally invasive surgical approaches for the treatment of thoracic cancers, including lung cancer, esophageal cancer, thymomas and thymic cancers, and malignant pleural mesothelioma.

Dr. Scott is a fellow of both the American College of Surgeons and the American College of Chest Physicians. He is a member of the Society of Thoracic Surgeons and the American Association for Thoracic Surgery. He serves as an editorial reviewer for a number of journals, including the Journal of

Thoracic and Cardiovascular Surgery, the Annals of Thoracic Surgery, Lung Cancer, and the Journal of Thoracic Oncology.

Dr. Scott serves as a member of the Thoracic Oncology Network of the American College of Chest Physicians. He is also a member of several national clinical trials groups, including the Eastern Cooperative Oncology Group, the Radiation Therapy Oncology Group, and the American College of Surgeons Oncology Group.

Dr. Scott received his medical degree from the University of Chicago Pritzker School of Medicine. He completed his general surgery residency and fellowship in cardiothoracic surgery at the University of Chicago Medical Center.

Consumer Health Titles from Addicus Books

Visit our online catalog at www.AddicusBooks.com

To Order Books:
Visit us online at: www.AddicusBooks.com
Call toll free: (800) 352-2873

For discounts on bulk purchases, call our Special Sales
Department at (402) 330-7493.
Or email us at: info@AddicusBooks.com

Addicus Books
P. O. Box 45327
Omaha, NE 68145

*Addicus Books is dedicated to publishing consumer health books
that comfort and educate.*